p53's Versatility in DNA Binding Site Recognition

SAYAN BHATTACHARJEE

Contents

Introduction 13
    THE GUARDIAN OF GENOME - p53 13
    THE GUARDIAN OF GENOME - p53 14
    TUMORIGENESIS... 14
    The structure of the p53 protein 15
    p53 REGULATIONS & FUNCTIONS 16
    p53 RESPONSE IN RESTING CELLS.. 18
    p53 RESPONSE IN STRESSED CELLS 18
    CELLULAR LOCALIZATION 19
    p53 MUTATION AND LOSS OF FUNCTION 20
    P152L MUTANT 22
    p53 AGGREGATION... 23
    PROTEIN DYNAMICITY AND FUNCTION 23
    p53 DYNAMICS... 24

Chapter – I... 25
    Fast time scale motion of p53DBD in complex with two different DNA complexes... 25
    Background:... 26

Objective:... 27
    Methodology:... 27
    NMR STUDIES 27
        Expression and Purification of p53 DBD:.. 27
        Oligo deoxynucleotide annealing:.. 28
        Titration Experiment: 29
        Preparation of p53-DBD-Oligonucleotide complex:.................................. 29
        Relaxation Dispersion: 29
        Nano-Pico second Dynamics:.. 29
        Data Processing:... 30
        Extraction of Relaxation Rates and NOE values:...................................... 30
        Estimation of Diffusion Tensor and Motional Parameters:...................... 31
    MD SIMULATION STUDIES 31
    Method: 31
        Analysis:... 32
        Root-mean-square Deviation (RMSD):... 32
        Root-mean-square Fluctuation (RMSF):... 32
        Solvent Accessible Surface Area (SASA):.. 33
        Principal Component Analysis (PCA):.. 33
        Dynamic Cross-Correlation Mapping (DCCM):....................................... 33
        Order Parameter (S^2) Calculation:.. 34
        Dynamic Path Analysis:... 34
    Results and Discussion 34
    NMR 34
        Chemical shift difference upon DNA binding:.. 34

Dynamic flexibility of p53-DBD: 36
MOLECULAR DYNAMICS: 37
Chapter - II 40
    Slow time scale motion in free and DNA-bound p53DBD: A comparison 40
    Background: 41
Objective: 42
    Methods: 42
        Sample preparation: 42
        NMR spectroscopy: 43
    Results and Discussion: 45
Chapter -III 52
    Electrostatic modulation in molecular recognition by p53 52
    Background: 53
Objective: 53
    Materials and Methods: 54
    MOLECULAR DYNAMICS 54
        Differential contact map and Dynamic cross correlation matrix (DCCM) 55
        Order parameter (S^2) 55
        Energy perturbation 56
        Energy network, construction of energy Hubs and shortest path 56
    Results and discussion 57
        Overall structure and dynamicity of p53DBD in complex with DNA or iASPP: 57
        Contributions of nonbonded interactions in p53DBD complexes with DNA and iASPP: 60
        Electrostatic energy reveals the evolutionarily conserved allosteric communication in the complexes: 69
        Pair-wise side-chain distance population shift modulates energy perturbations and manipulates side-chain conformational entropy: 75
Chapter - IV 79
    Structural and functional characterization of both full-length wild type and P152L p53 79
Background and Objective 80
Materials and Methods 80
    Expression and Purification of FL-p53: 80
    Atomic force microscopy (AFM): 80
    Transmission electron microscopy (TEM): 80
    Cryogenic electron microscopy (Cryo-EM): 81
    Dynamic light scattering (DLS): 81
    Denaturation experiment: 81
    Isothermal Titration Calorimetry (ITC): 82
    Results and Discussion: 82
References 87

Introduction

THE GUARDIAN OF GENOME - p53

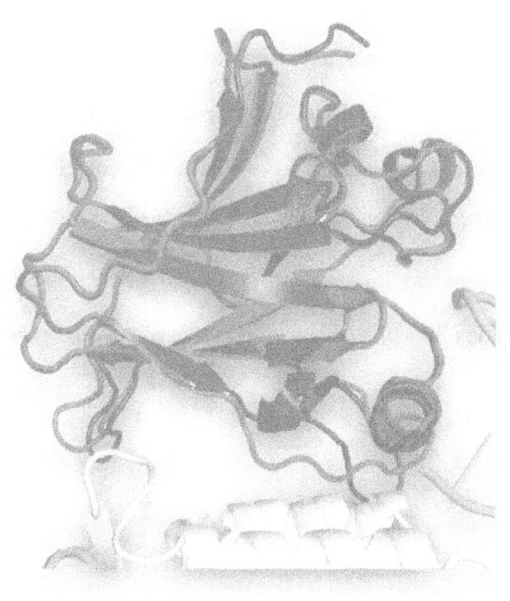

THE GUARDIAN OF GENOME - p53

The human body consists of innumerable cells that provide structure and carry out specialized functions. Some of the cells present in the tissues divide, generate new cells, and replace worn-out cells with new ones. This process is normally strictly regulated by built-in controls. Loss of these controls may cause the cells to proliferate abnormally. One of the central players in maintaining proper regulation of cell growth is the tumor suppressor protein p53.

TUMORIGENESIS

Currently, cancer represents a major global health concern, not to mention the huge economic burden.[1] Tumor progression is a complex multi-step process that is dictated by a series of genetic or epigenetic events that alter the genomic DNA. These may include mutations, deletions, chromosomal translocation, amplification, histone modification, DNA methylation, etc, affecting the expression of genes responsible for maintaining homeostasis.[2] The common properties that are required by a normal cell to evade the anti-cancer defense mechanism and transform into a cancerous one include self-sufficiency in growth signals, insensitivity to anti-growth signals, evasion of programmed cell death, limitless replicative potential, sustained angiogenesis and finally tumor invasion and metastasis.[3] These are accompanied by activation of oncogenes, inactivation of tumor suppressor genes like p53 as well as suppression of DNA repair systems.

The structure of the p53 protein

p53, commonly known as the 'Guardian of the Genome', is responsible for protecting genome integrity.[4,5] It was originally discovered in 1979, in complex with the large T-antigen of tumor virus Simian Virus 40 (SV-40),[6,7] but its role as a tumor suppressor was established only after 1989.[8,9] It is encoded by the TP53 gene located on the short arm of chromosome 17 (17p13) of human (GenBank Accession Number: NC_000017.10). The gene has two promoters, one upstream of exon 1 and another internal promoter in intron 4.[10] Full-length p53 is transcribed by the P1 promoter present upstream of exon 1.[11] Human p53 is a 393 amino acid long protein with a molecular weight of 43.7 kDa that has been conserved during evolution.[12] The gene consists of 11 exons, where the first one is non-coding, with five highly conserved regions encoded by exon 2 to exon 8 that are crucial for p53 functions.[13,14]

The protein consists of six domains, whose molecular characterization has revealed numerous interacting partners as well as post-translational regulatory sites.

- Transactivation domain (TAD): Residues 1 to 42 – regulates several pro-apoptotic genes.[15]
- Proline-rich domain (PRD): Residues 64 to 92 - Important for apoptotic activity and repression of target genes.[16]
- DNA binding domain (DBD): Residues 92 to 292 – The DNA binding region, pivotal for p53 transcriptional activity.[17]
- Nuclear localization signaling domain (NLSD): Residues 316 to 325 – Crucial for the nuclear localization of the protein.[18]
- Oligomerization domain (OD): Residues 307 to 355 – Essential for p53 tetramerization. p53 forms highly symmetrical tetramers, dimers of two homodimers that are crucial for transactivation and growth suppression.[19]

- C-terminal domain (CTD): Residues 356 to 393 – Responsible for DNA-binding downregulation, DNA-damage recognition, transcriptional regulation and also implicated in apoptosis.[20]

p53, as a tetramer, can recognize[21] and bind to a wide range of DNA sequences, commonly known as response elements (RE). The DNA-binding domain (DBD) of p53 acts as a clamp that binds to the varied DNA REs. Structurally, the DBD consists of a β-sandwich formed of 9 strands in 2 sheets with a Greek-key topology. It readily recognizes the 10 bp consensus sequence 5'-PuPuPuC(A/T)(T/A)GPyPyPy-3' present in two copies, separated by a 0-13 bp in the regulatory region of the target gene promoter.[22] p53 binding to DNA may recruit transcriptional co-regulators that help control target gene expression. Thus, it regulates a wide range of target genes either by transcriptional activation or by modulating other protein activities by direct association. By modulating different transcriptional targets, p53 responds to cellular damage and prevents the propagation of damaged cells.

p53 REGULATIONS & FUNCTIONS

p53 influences various cellular functions by both transcription-dependent as well as independent pathways. Most p53 activated promoter genes contain consensus sequences.[22] Functions of p53 target genes include cell cycle arrest, DNA repair, apoptosis, senescence, angiogenesis, and metastasis. p53, when activated, has the ability to modify cell fate (life or death), either by inducing cell cycle arrest or by forcing it to commit suicide, i.e. activation of programmed cell death.[23,24] This makes it absolutely crucial to regulate the p53 concentration and activation in normal undamaged cells. This regulation can be achieved both at the protein as well as mRNA levels.[25] However, different cellular stresses can induce multiple post-translational modifications including phosphorylation, acetylation, sumoylation, glycosylation, or ubiquitination that in turn modulates its stability, DNA-binding, transactivation and transcriptional activity.[26]

Other important functions of p53 include DNA repair, inhibition of angiogenesis, senescence response to short telomeres, inflammation, stem cell renewal and differentiation, neurodegeneration, aging, embryo development regulation of metabolism and autophagy.[27,28] Recently, p53 has also been shown to control the expression of various microRNAs.[29]

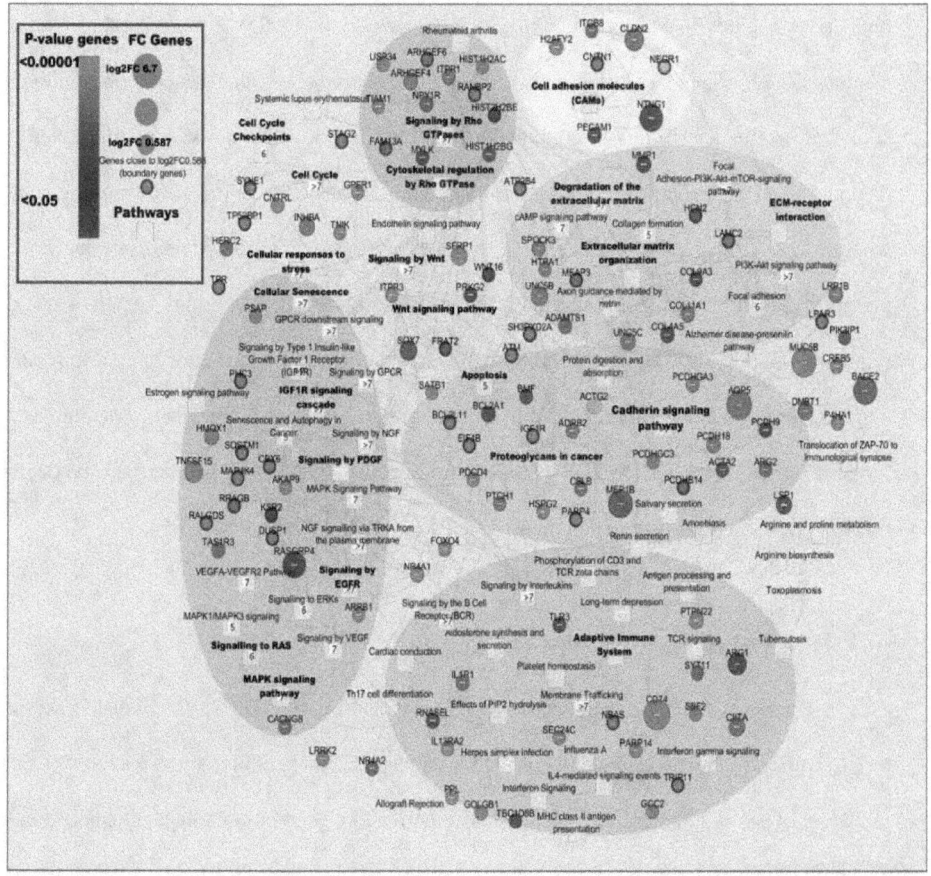

Figure 1. Network of pathways and genes induced by P152L p53 expression: RNA-seq analysis of the tumor (P152Lp53 vs Control) showing the pathways and genes upregulated (fold

change ≥ 1.5, p value ≥ 0.05). Some of the boundary gene (fold change ≥ 1.41 but <1.5) are also considered in the pathway network

p53 RESPONSE IN RESTING CELLS

In resting cells, p53 regulates cell cycle progression. It is also responsible for genomic stability and a major deciding factor of apoptosis. Under normal conditions, p53 is present at lower levels in unstressed cells. Its action is regulated by MDM2, also referred to as HDM2 in humans, that binds to p53 and marking it for degradation.[30] MDM2 binds to the N-terminal residues 17-27 of p53, in the vicinity of TAD, a region containing several phosphorylation sites.[31] It acts as an E3 ligase, conjugating ubiquitin to p53, thus marking it for proteasomal degradation. It then shuttles the ubiquitin-p53 complex back to the cytoplasm from the nucleus, where it is degraded.[32] The transcription of the MDM2 gene is, in turn, regulated by p53. The promoter has a p53-binding motif, and thus higher p53 concentrations generate an auto-regulatory loop.[33] This regulatory circuit helps maintain a rapid turnover of the p53 protein and allowing it to be functionally active only for a short duration upon appropriate signaling. Several proteins cooperate with MDM2 in its regulation of p53. Additionally, p53 can also be degraded independently by two other protein ligases COP1 and Pirh-1.[34]

p53 RESPONSE IN STRESSED CELLS

A pre-requisite for stabilization of p53 is inhibition of MDM2, which can be achieved through different independent pathways. DNA damage or other cellular stress responses (such as radiation, hypoxia, telomere erosion, oncogene activation, genotoxic damage, chemotherapeutic agents, etc.) that affect normal cell division, activates p53 leading to its rapid accumulation in the stressed cells. This activation may be achieved by p53 phosphorylation by its upstream DNA damage-induced kinases.[35] Activation can also be achieved by N-terminal phosphorylation by stress-activated protein kinases such as DNA-PK (DNA-dependent protein kinase) that is activated by DNA damage.[10] Additionally, phosphorylation of MDM2 also disrupts the p53-MDM2 interaction.[36] C-terminal phosphorylation by CDKs, PKCs, and others also mediated the sequence-specific binding of p53.[37] p53 can also be stabilized by deubiquitination by p53-associated factor HAUSP. p53 activation disrupts the p53-Mdm2 complex, inhibiting ubiquitin-mediated p53 degradation, resulting in unbound p53 that is now free to bind the desired target genes. p53 then undergoes extensive modifications that modulate its stability, cellular localization, and interaction with other proteins. The potential outcomes of p53 activation can be varied including cell cycle arrest, DNA repair, apoptosis, senescence, differentiation, inhibition of angiogenesis or metastasis[38], and are determined by multiple factors including interacting partners or co-regulators, activation stimuli, modification state of p53, etc. Alternatively, phosphorylation of p53 by HIPK2 dissociates it from the p53-MDM2 complex and induces apoptosis.[39] Other modifications include acetylation of the C-terminal lysine by histone acetyltransferases like p300/CBP or methylation by methyltransferases that may enhance apoptosis or senescence.[39,40]

Depending on the severity of the damage, p53 can stall the cell cycle progress and sequester the cells either before DNA replication in the G1 phase or before mitosis in the G2 phase or at the G1/S regulation point. The cell cycle arrest allows time for repair of the lesion. In case of irreparable damage, the cells are eliminated from the system by p53-activated apoptotic (programmed cell death) pathway, thus preventing the proliferation of damaged cells that are more likely to exhibit abnormal cell growth.

CELLULAR LOCALIZATION

The shuttle of p53 between the nucleus and cytoplasm of a cell is tightly regulated and is determined by the nuclear localization signals (NLS) as well as the nuclear export signals (NES).[18,41] p53 has three NLS sequences that, upon receipt of the desired stimuli, enable nuclear transport required for p53-mediated transcriptional regulation.[41] The NLS sequences bind selective receptors and allow the passage of p53 through the nuclear pore complex.[42] The NES is a highly conserved region and sufficient for efficient nuclear export.[43] This is necessary for efficient degradation. An N-terminal NES consists of 2 sites that are phosphorylated following DNA damage, thus inhibiting the nuclear export of p53, resulting in its enhanced activity.[44] Additionally, efficient export to the cytoplasm requires the ubiquitin ligase function of MDM2.[45]

p53 MUTATION AND LOSS OF FUNCTION

The importance of p53 mutations in tumor cell biology is irrefutable. p53 dysfunction, either due to mutation or loss of expression, is the most common denominator in all human cancers.[46] Wild-type p53 mediates important functions such as regulation of the cell cycle and programmed cell death. Deficiency of p53 function, created by mutation or modifications, abrogates normal cell cycle checkpoints and apoptosis, generating a favorable milieu for genomic instability and carcinogenesis.

In nature, 80% of these p53 alterations are caused by missense mutations leading to functionally altered p53.[46] Though the mutations are distributed over all the coding exons, there is a strong predominance in exons 5-8, encoding the DNA binding domain, making the DBD of p53 highly prone to mutations, and these mutations have been implicated in most cancers. Further, 90% of these mutations occur within residues 110-290 of the sequence-specific DNA-binding core domain, commonly known as the hot spot region, thus rendering p53 transcriptionally inactive.[47] The six most common hotspot mutations include – R175, R245, R248, R249, R273, and R282.

The mutations can be divided into two groups –

- Group I mutations that include the most frequently occurring mutations. These affect p53 DNA-binding without affecting the wild-type conformation.

- Group II mutations include conformationally altered p53 conferring more severe phenotype.[48]

Missense mutations in the DBD can have at least three different consequences – loss of DNA contact, a local perturbation in the domain structure, or unfolding of the entire domain, resulting in partial or complete loss of p53 binding to target genes.[47] This hampers the p53 mediated cellular response to stress signals. Additionally, they also interfere with any residual wild type (wt) p53. Furthermore, they are also involved in causing resistance to common anti-cancer therapies that directly or indirectly rely on activation of p53-mediated apoptosis.[49] Such mutations very often result in elevated levels of the mutated protein, probably due to loss of inhibition by negative feedback loops.

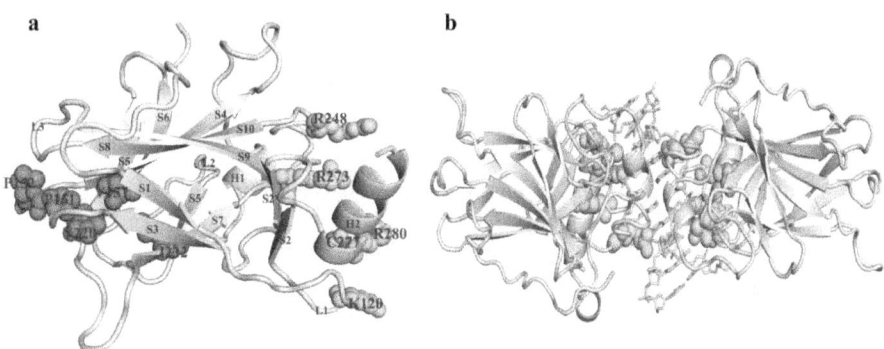

Figure 2. Secondary structure of p53-DBD. (a) Monomeric wt-DBD. Magenta spheres represent the allosteric residues mutated frequently and **(b)** Dimeric wt-DBD. Green spheres are the DNA binding residue.

These cancer mutants provide a highly specific drug target. If the mutated domain can somehow with treatment be induced to take up the wild-type conformation, p53 functions including apoptosis can be restored. Additionally, this shift to the wild-type conformation will also eliminate any gain of functions of the mutants. This will help in selectively eliminating mutant containing cancerous cells, without causing harm to the normal cells expressing wt p53.

There is also a fraction of mutations that occur outside the DNA-binding domain, including the transactivation and oligomerization domain.

p53 inactivation and loss of function can also occur via non-mutational mechanisms. Overexpression of p53 negative regulators like MDM2 is also a common phenomenon in various tumors. The over-expression of MDM2 leads to enhanced degradation of p53, rendering the cells in an effective p53-null condition. In these situations, disruption of the p53-MDM2 complex is critical for the activation of p53. However, inactivation of an upstream modulator executing this process has also been observed in certain tumors. Mutation in upstream p53 kinases like DNA damage-induced kinases results in unphosphorylated p53, thus rendering it inactive.[50]

Appropriate subcellular localization is also crucial for the regulation of p53 functions. Mutations in the C-terminal lysine residues abrogate MDM2-mediated p53 ubiquitination, thus hampering its nuclear export.[51] Loss of p53 function is often associated with its failure to accumulate in the nucleus in some types of tumors. This may be due to hyperactivity of MDM2 or cytoplasmic sequestration of p53 in complex with glucocorticoid receptors (GR).[52]

P152L MUTANT

The mutant contains a leucine at position 152, residing in the S3/S4 turn opposite the DNA binding surface of the DBD, replacing the wild-type Proline. Though the mutant can efficiently tetramerize, the DNA binding by the full-length protein is lost. However, the DBD individually can bind to DNA.

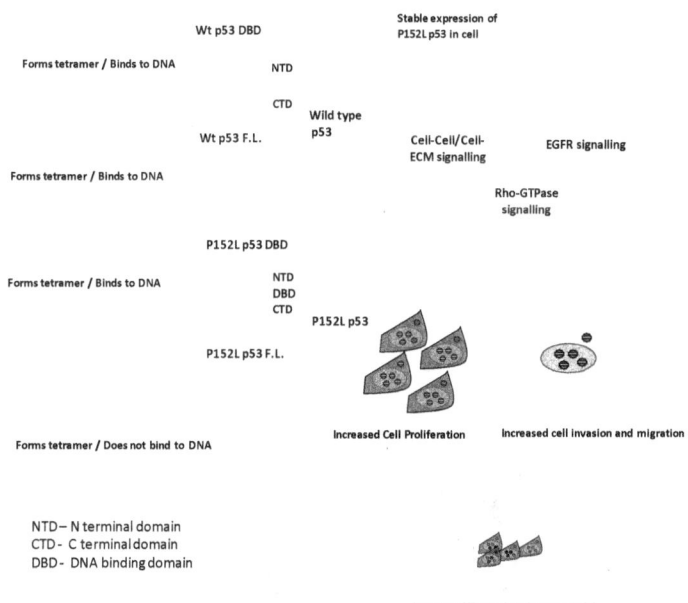

Figure 3. Summarized cartoon representation of the biochemical and functional characterisation of P152L p53.

p53 AGGREGATION

p53 has low thermodynamic stability. Mutations in the protein can make it prone to aggregation because of lower structural stabilities of the core domain.[53] Aggregation of p53 mutants can lead to dominant-negative and gain-of-function effects that increase cancer aggressiveness and progression.[54]

PROTEIN DYNAMICITY AND FUNCTION

Dynamicity of a protein defines the fluctuations within a stable protein molecule without external perturbations. Proteins are responsible for a repertoire of functions within a living cell, and these biological functions are primarily dependent on their 3D structure. However, these structures are dynamic, giving rise to multiple conformations, with each conformation playing different roles.[55] Conformational dynamics play a pivotal role in molecular recognition, enzyme catalysis, and allosteric modulations.[56] Thus, understanding protein dynamics provides a better knowledge of protein functions.

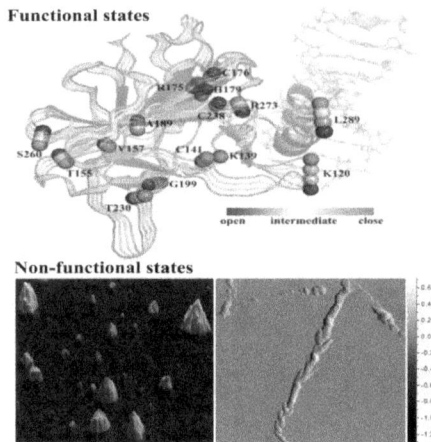

Figure 4. Conformational states. Functional states are shown by principal components of 1μs simulation where spheres represent NMR dispersion (μs-ms). Non-functional states i.e. oligomers (left) and Fibril (right) of P152L mutant of p53, are indicated by AFM images.

p53 DYNAMICS

Despite intense research over the years and the well-known impact of p53 on cancer, no drugs have been developed to combat this deadly disease that currently inflicts millions worldwide. p53 being a versatile protein with complex cellular functions, much remains to be probed into, to get a clear understanding, with one such factor being the dynamicity of the protein.

Chapter – I

Fast time scale motion of p53DBD in complex with two different DNA complexes

Background:

Transcription factor p53, a tumor suppressor protein, is inactivated and degraded by MDM2 (a negative regulator) in normal cells. DNA damage or stress (e.g., UV, chemical agents, oxidative stress, etc.) induce disruption of the p53-MDM2 complex, leading to elevation of concentration and activation of p53. Once activated, it can either promote cell cycle arrest (at G1/S checkpoint) to allow DNA repair or bring about apoptosis.

p53 consists of six domains:

1. Transactivation domain (TAD): Residues 1 to 42
2. Proline rich domain (PRD): Residues 43 to 63
3. DNA-binding domain (DBD): Residues 92 to 292
4. Nuclear localization signaling domain (NLSD): Residues 316 to 325
5. Oligomerization domain (OD): Residues 307 to 355
6. C-terminal domain (CTD): Residues 356 to 393

Among these domains, only the DBD binds to consensus sequences of DNA. Two decameric half-sites RRRCWWGYYY (R = A, G; W = A, T; Y = C, T), separated by 0-13 base pairs, form the consensus sequences.[22] p53 binds to each decameric half-sites as a dimer, and each dimer forms a tetramer (dimer of dimer).

There are hundreds of such specific sequences in the human genome recognized by DBD of p53. The main goal of this project is to find out how a single DBD recognizes this wide range of variation, either by conformational changes or by other factors, such as protein dynamics. We plan to calculate conformational entropies upon binding with different DNA sequences that will be calculated, which will provide the idea of the role of entropy in DNA recognition. In about half of all human cancers, p53 is inactivated by mutation. Maximum mutations are found in the DNA-binding domain. A subset of these mutations also gains other growth-promoting properties, and these mutants are called gain-of-function (GOF) mutants.[57] Tumors that harbor these GOF alleles are in general drug-resistant and aggressive, making it clinically relevant to understand the properties of GOF-p53 proteins. It is assumed that these gains of functions are through structural perturbations Induced by the mutations. Allosteric crosstalk is a very effective mechanism for a protein to be activated in most of the physiological processes, such as Response Element (RE) recognition, metabolism, and catalysis.[58] Allostery plays a crucial role for a protein to adopt several conformational states with different activities. Specific binding of a protein to multiple REs, is sometimes accomplished by selectively stabilizing a particular conformational state, thereby diversifying its activity.

Objective:

In this chapter, I have elucidated allosteric communication path between the active site of the wild type DNA binding domain (wt DBD) of p53 with those allosteric regions that are highly prone to be mutated, consequently losing the binding affinity to DNA. I have used NMR spectroscopy and MD simulation to characterize residue-specific dynamicity changes as well as the allosteric signal transfer of "the guardian of the genome" upon binding to two different REs.

Methodology:

In this section the difference in dynamics of the DBD of wild-type p53 upon binding with two different DNA response elements was characterized.

NMR STUDIES

Expression and Purification of p53 DBD:

Protein-specific plasmids were transformed into *E. coli* Rosetta cells through the heat shock method in brief 5ml of bacterial culture at OD 0.6 was washed and placed at 4°C in 50μl $CaCl_2$ solution for 30 minutes. Plasmid was added to it and heated in a water bath to 42°C for 45 seconds and then placed to 4°C. 900 μl of LB media was added to it and left 1 hour for shaking at 37°C.[59] Transformed screened cells were then grown in 2 ml of LB-media with 100 μg/ml carbenicillin (stock in water) for 8 h at 37°C. 500 μl of this culture was then added to 2 ml of unlabeled M9 minimal medium containing the same concentration of antibiotic and grown overnight at similar temperature conditions. 2 ml of this minimal media culture was then added to an equal volume of modified M9 minimal medium in 99% D_2O supplemented with ^{15}N labeled 1 g/L $^{15}NH_4Cl$ and 4 g/L ^{13}C-glucose and grown for ~ 8 h. The culture was centrifuged at 500 rcf at room temperature for 10 min. The pellet was washed with D_2O containing modified M9 minimal media to remove any residual traces of water and re-dissolved in a 500 μl MM-D_2O to make a complete homogeneous solution. This is then added to 2 ml of M9-99% D_2O medium and grown overnight. The final culture was grown the next day at 37°C, 180 rpm till the cell density reaches OD_{600} of 0.8, followed by induction with 1 mM IPTG at 18°C for 18 h. Cells were pelleted down at 6000 rcf for 10 mins at 4°C and resuspended in 20 mM potassium phosphate pH 6.8, 50 mM potassium chloride and 5mM DTT and sonicated on ice (25% duty cycle, 80% amplitude) followed by ultracentrifugation at 91,000 rcf at 4°C for 1 h. Protein purification was done with HiTrap SP HP cation exchange column in AKTA FPLC with phosphate buffer and 500 mM NaCl. Purification was confirmed with 12.5% SDS PAGE.

Oligodeoxynucleotide annealing:

Duplex oligonucleotides containing selected p53 response elements were designed such that p53 can bind as a dimer. Two such sequences (DNA-A: 5'-GGGCATGCCC-3' and its complementary sequence, DNA-B: 5'-GGACATGTCC-3' and its complementary sequence) were used for NMR studies. For annealing experiments, each strand was dissolved in 20 mM Potassium Phosphate buffer of pH 6.8 in salt 150 mM NaCl without DTT, mixed at an equal molar ratio, heated to 90°C, and allowed to cool down at room temperature. To check for proper annealing NOESY NMR spectra was acquired.

Titration Experiment:

^{2}H, ^{15}N labeled p53-DBD was added in four successive steps to DNA, and after each addition, TROSY-HSQC was acquired at 18°C to monitor the peak shift upon binding. Finally, 25% of excess oligonucleotide duplex was added to ensure complete binding. In each step of titration, the molar ratio of p53-DBD to duplex oligonucleotide was 2:1.

Preparation of p53-DBD-Oligonucleotide complex:

P53-DBD and oligonucleotides were mixed at a 2:1 molar ratio followed by incubation at room temperature for 30 minutes and then kept in ice for 1 h. Final concentration and volume of ^{2}H, ^{15}N labeled p53-DBD was 290 µM and 200 µl, respectively.

Relaxation Dispersion:

For measuring the p53-DBD backbone dynamics upon binding to different DNA sequences, relaxation dispersion NMR experiments were performed in an interleaved manner, acquiring multiple 2D {^{15}N, ^{2}H} spectra. The acquisition time for each {^{15}N, ^{2}H} spectrum was 44 ms (*t1*) x 83 ms (*t2*). The proton carrier was set at 4.7 ppm corresponding to the water resonance, while the ^{15}N carrier frequency was set to 118.5 ppm. ^{15}N quadrature detection was done with the echo-anti-echo method during *t1* evolution. These experiments were typically employed with the pulse sequences with gradient and sensitivity enhanced techniques recruiting flip-back and 3-9-19 binomial pulses for water suppression.

Nano-Pico second Dynamics:

Backbone amide ^{15}N spin-lattice relaxation (R_1), rotating frame relaxation ($R_{1\rho}$) dispersion experiments, and the steady-state heteronuclear {^{1}H}-^{15}N NOE measurements were performed following the pulse schemes developed by Lakomek *et al*. The experiments were acquired at 18°C on Bruker Avance III 700 MHz (16.47 T field) spectrometer equipped with a 5 mm cryogenic probe with a z-axis gradient magnetic field capability. For measuring ^{15}N the spin-lattice relaxation rate constants (R_1), the dispersion measurement experiments were performed by acquiring a series of 7 interleaved spectra with pseudo-randomized longitudinal relaxation delays of 0, 240, 440, 80, 320, 160 and 600 ms. Similarly, the rotating frame relaxation rate constants ($R_{1\rho}$) were estimated from the dispersion measurements performed by acquiring an equal number of interleaved spectra with the pseudo-randomized relaxation delays 5, 80, 1, 20, 40, 10 and 120 ms. A recycle delay of two seconds was set for R_1 and $R_{1\rho}$ measurement. The heteronuclear {^{1}H}-^{15}N NOE experiments were performed with a 5 s presaturation delay after 1 s recycle delay for the NOE spectrum whereas in the reference spectrum 4 s recycle delay was used without any presaturation pulse. The total number of complex points acquired in the *t1* x *t2* dimension was 144 x 1280 in all the experiments for each interleaved spectrum.

Data Processing:

All NMR spectra were processed with the NMRPipe program.[60] Visualization and spectral assignments of the p53-DNA complex were done using Sparky.[61] A Lorentzian-to-Gaussian multiplication window was applied to the FIDs prior to Fourier transformation to process all the spectra. The peaks were fitted to a Gaussian line shape using nLinLS sub-routine in NMRPipe.

Extraction of Relaxation Rates and NOE values:

The peak intensities were extracted and the trajectories of peak intensities were plotted against relaxation delays. Fitting the peak intensities to a single exponential function helped to extract the residue-specific relaxation rates for R_1 and $R_{1\rho}$. The {^{1}H}-^{15}N NOE values were calculated from the ratio of peak intensities between the spectra acquired with or without presaturation pulses. The root-mean square (r.m.s.) spectral noise obtained from NMRPipe was used to estimate the errors R_1, $R_{1\rho}$, and NOE. The transverse (R_2) relaxation rates were then calculated as a function of R_1, $R_{1\rho}$ rates as well as spin-lock field and ^{15}N frequency offset.

Estimation of Diffusion Tensor and Motional Parameters:

The $r2r1\_tm^{62}$ program developed by Dr. Arthur G. Palmer (Columbia University) was used to estimate the rotational correlation time (τ_c). The initial estimation of τ_c was made from the R_2/R_1 ratio as input. The τ_c thus obtained was then used as the input for the estimation of rotational diffusion tensor using the program $r2r1\_diffusion$, developed by Tjandra et al.[63,64] The calculation also utilizes the PDB structure of the protein as input, along with the rotational correlation time. The PDB structure must be translated and rotated appropriately to locate the center of mass with the origin and align the moment of inertia with the Cartesian axes. This was achieved by using pdbinertia.[65] Before translation and rotation of the PDB structure, protons were added using WHATIF server. The diffusion tensor estimate was used as the input for an initial round of Lipari–Szabo model-free analysis followed by the simultaneous optimization of both the diffusion tensor and model-free parameters. This was accomplished by iterating the FASTModelfree[66] code used in Modelfree[67] software until a self-consistent set of parameters was obtained. The N–H bond length and ^{15}N CSA used for the calculation were 1.015 Å and −179 ppm, respectively.

MD SIMULATION STUDIES

Molecular Dynamics simulations of the three wild-type p53 DBD-RE complexes were performed at pH 6.8, with temperature 18°C under 1 bar pressure with *AMBER99sb* force field[68] using GROMACS v5.1.2 software package.[69]

Method:

Crystal structure of the DNA-bound dimeric DBD of wild-type p53 with corresponding PDB IDs of 2AC0, 2ADY abbreviated as DNA-A, DNA-B, respectively were selected for MD simulations. Dimeric p53 DBD-DNA complexes were obtained from available tetrameric complexes. At the same time, crystallographic waters present in the structures were removed using PyMOL. For correlating with NMR experimental conditions, the pH of all complexes was adjusted by protonating required residues based on pK_a values, obtained from the PROPKA framework of PDB2PQR web server.[70] Solvation was done by the TIP3P water model[71] followed by neutralizing the overall charge with 150 mM NaCl within a cubic box with cut off distances of 1 nm between the complex surfaces and the edges of the box. The energy minimized systems were equilibrated in an NVT followed by NPT condition by restraining positions for 1 ns. A final simulation was carried out for up to 400 ns in triplicates, and trajectories were stored at every 50 ps interval.

Analysis:

Data corresponding to all trajectories were analyzed by different GROMACS v5.1.2 tools. In this analysis only the protein dimers were included, excluding the DNA by making proper index through *g_make_ndx* tool.

Root-mean-square Deviation (RMSD):

Root-mean-square deviation, based on the backbone and side-chain atoms, was calculated using the *g_rmsdist* tool for all the triplicate datasets, and the mean and standard deviation were calculated to determine the proper energy minimization and stabilization of the structures.

Root-mean-square Fluctuation (RMSF):

Root-mean-square fluctuation for the Cα atom of each residue was calculated separately for each simulation set using the *g_rmsf* tool. The average residue-specific values and standard deviations were calculated over the triplicate datasets for relative comparison of the fluctuation between two complexes.

Solvent Accessible Surface Area (SASA):

Surface area based on hydrophobic and hydrophilic accessibility over the 400 ns simulation was calculated for the protein dimer excluding the DNA molecule using g_sas tool, to monitor the change in conformation on residue basis over time throughout the trajectory.

Principal Component Analysis (PCA):

Principal Component Analysis was done by calculating the covariance matrix of the atomic fluctuations based on the Cα atom. Diagonalization of this matrix gives a set of eigenvectors and eigenvalues, which describe different modes of fluctuations of the protein. The eigenvectors corresponding to the largest eigenvalues i.e., "principal components," were analyzed by g_covar and g_anaeig tools provided by GROMACS based on the 400 ns trajectories of the three complexes.

Dynamic Cross-Correlation Mapping (DCCM):

Dynamic Cross-Correlation Mapping was analyzed based on all and C-alpha atoms to measure the extent of atomic fluctuations of the protein complex and correlated with one another on a residue basis. Here the correlation is scored by 1 and that of the anti-correlation case is -1.[72]

$$C_{ij} = \frac{\langle (r_i - \langle r_i \rangle)(r_j - \langle r_j \rangle) \rangle}{\sqrt{(\langle r_i^2 \rangle - \langle r_i \rangle^2)(\langle r_j^2 \rangle - \langle r_j \rangle^2)}}$$

Where i and j correspond to any two atoms, residues, or domains; r_i and r_j are position vectors of i and j; and the angle brackets denote an ensemble average. Interatomic cross-correlation fluctuations between any two pairs of atoms (or residues) can be calculated by using this expression and can be represented graphically by the DCCM. The value of C_{ij} can vary from -1 (completely anti-correlated motion) to +1 (completely correlated motion).

Order Parameter (S^2) Calculation:

BackboneN-H vectors were selected to calculate S^2 over the period of trajectory, which represent dynamicity of protein with the value 1 indicates complete rigidity and towards 0 represents enhanced dynamicity.

$$S^2 = \frac{1}{2}(3\sum_{i=1}^{3}\sum_{j=1}^{3}\langle\langle\mu_i\mu_j\rangle^2 - 1\rangle$$

in which µ1, µ2, and µ3 are the x, y, and z components of the relevant bond vector scaled to unit magnitude, µ, respectively.[96] Angular brackets indicate averaging over the snapshots.

Dynamic Path Analysis:

To monitor the connectivity of neighboring residues as well as the allosteric crosstalk between different residues, betweenness and community clustering was done based on those having any heavy atom within 4.5 Å for greater than 75% of the simulation and strong correlation within value ± 0.8 to ±1 of DCCM.

Results and Discussion

NMR

Chemical shift difference upon DNA binding:

The changes in the local protein conformation upon binding to DNA were estimated from the changes in residue-specific amide chemical shift **(Figure 1)** ($\Delta\delta_{amide}$)

$$\Delta\delta_{amide} = \sqrt{(\Delta\delta_{HN})^2 + (\Delta\delta_{N}/5)^2}$$

Local perturbations were observed at DNA binding loop L1, helix H2 and loop L3. Significantly the dimerization interface helix H1 shows significant chemical shift change with respect to the free p53 chemical shift. Note that both the complexes show similar kind of chemical shift pattern, although there are significant quantitative differences. The results imply the formation of the dimeric p53-DBD-DNA complexes.

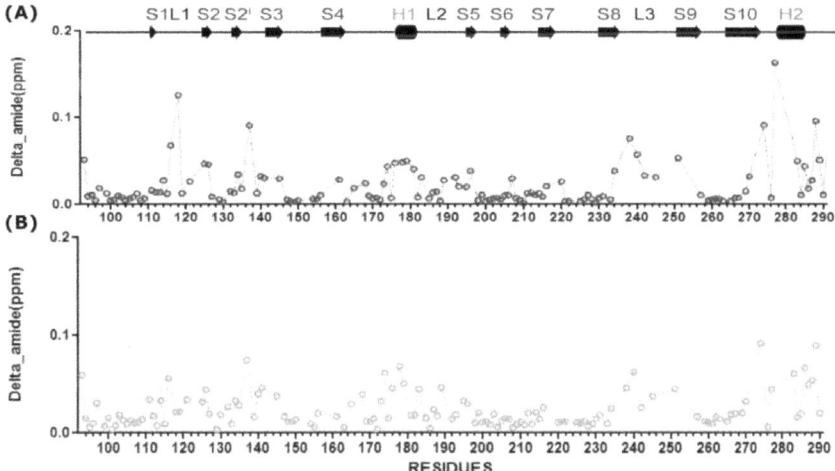

Figure 1.Comparison of conformational difference between free p53-DBD and bound p53-DBD with two different DNA REs. Residue specific delta amide shift for (A) p53DBD-DNA-A complex (B) p53DBD-DNA-B complex.

To focus on the difference in local conformation changes between two different complexes, a delta-amide difference between p53-DBD-DNA-A and p53-DBD-DNA-B complex was calculated **(Figure 2)**. Differences in chemical shifts in both complexes were found in loop L1 and helix H2.

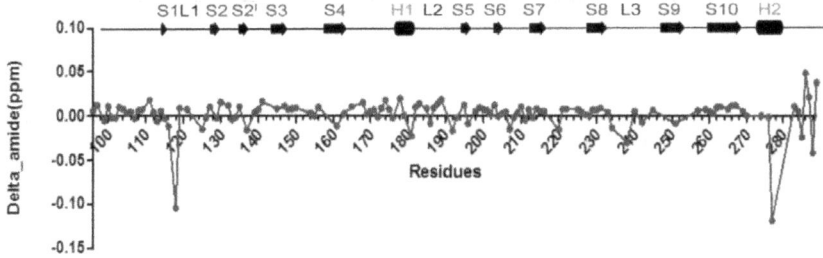

Figure 2. Local conformational change of p53DBD in two different complexes. Residue specific Delta amide difference between p53DBD in p53DBD_DNA-A and p53-DBD_DNA-B complexes.

Dynamic flexibility of p53-DBD:

The ratio of relaxation parameters R_2/R_1 indicates the conformational flexibility occurring in both the fast time-scale (ps-ns range) and the slow time-scale (μs-ms range). The values of R_2/R_1 beyond the positive SD from the mean value correspond to the residues fluctuating in slow time-scale motion and that with lower values than the negative SD from the mean value corresponds to residues with fast time-scale motion. The rotational correlation times (τ_m) were found to be 15.8 ± 0.1 ns for perdeuterated free p53-DBD, 28.8 ± 0.1 ns for p53-DBD-DNA-A and 28.1 ± 0.1 ns for p53-DBD-DNA-B complex, suggesting the formation of a dimer in presence of DNA sequences **(Figure 3)**.

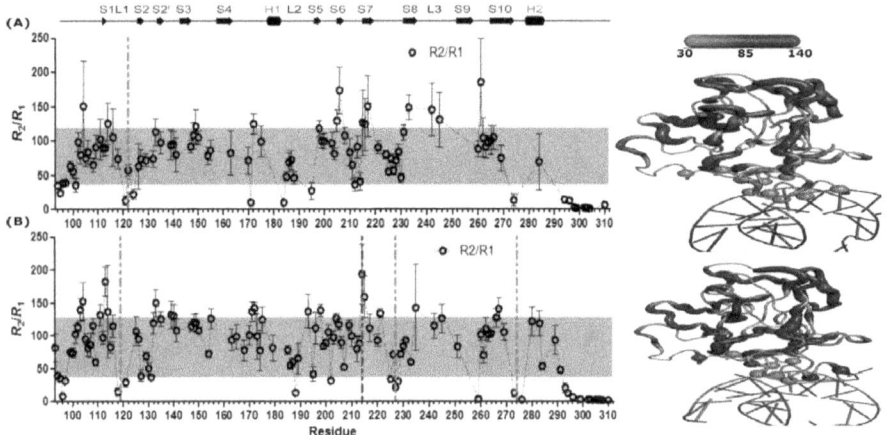

Figure 3. Timescale dependent dynamicity difference. R_2/R_1 values of p53-DBD with (A) DNA-A and (B) DNA-B as complex. Residue specific R_2/R_1 values are mapped in 3D structures [pdb id: 2ADY for (A) and pdb id: 2AC0 for (B)] and red to blue colour scheme applied where red means low and blue means high R2/R1 ratio i.e. red is fast time scale dynamics and blue is slow time scale dynamics. Spheres are indicating the DNA binding

residues of p53. Red and blue dashed lines indicate the regions with significant difference in R_2/R_1 values in two complexes.

MOLECULAR DYNAMICS:

Residue specific C-alpha RMSF shows a significant difference in loop L1, helix H2 to loop L2, and in loop containing residues from Y220 to T230 in two different complexes (**Figure 4**).

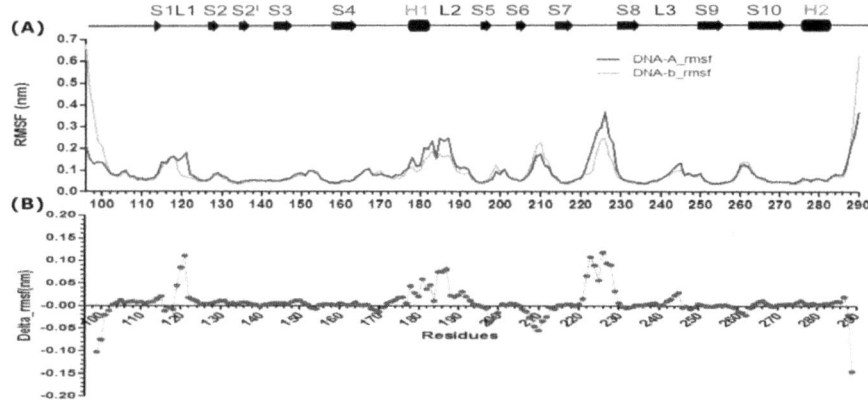

Figure 4: Fast time scale residue specific motion based on 400ns MD simulation. (A) AverageRMSF from three different simulation based on C-alpha atom of p53-DBD with DNA-A and DNA-B as complex (B) Difference in RMSF between p53-DBD with DNA-A and DNA-B as complex.

Backbone N-H vector-based order parameter of the p53-DBD complex with DNA-A and DNA-B shows remarkable changes in loop L1, helix H2 to loop L2, and loop consisting of residues from Y220 to T230. This is consistent with RMSF values based on the C-alpha atom, and that of NMR derived relaxation parameters (**Figure 5**).

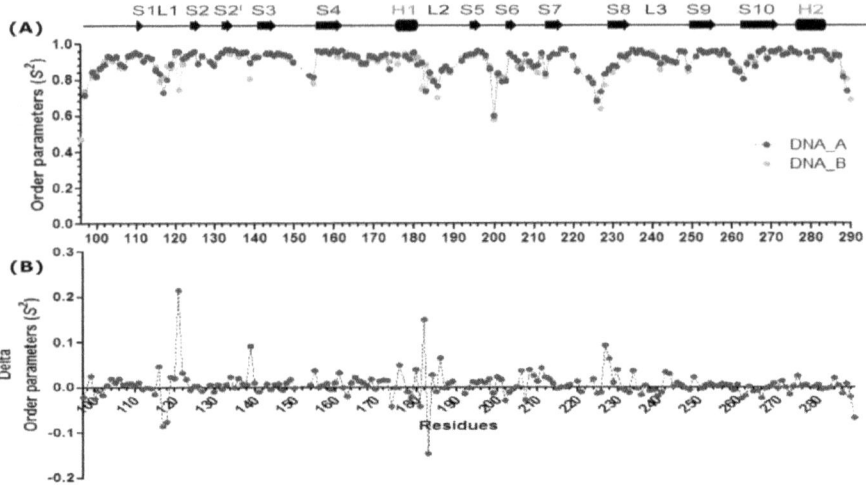

Figure 5: Backbone dynamic fluctuation based on 400ns MD simulation. (A) Residue specific order parameter comparison (B) difference between order parameter of p53-DBD in two protein DNA complexes.

All-atom correlation throughout the trajectory has been calculated to establish the possible allosteric connectivity and analysis of the path of correlation (**Figure 6**).

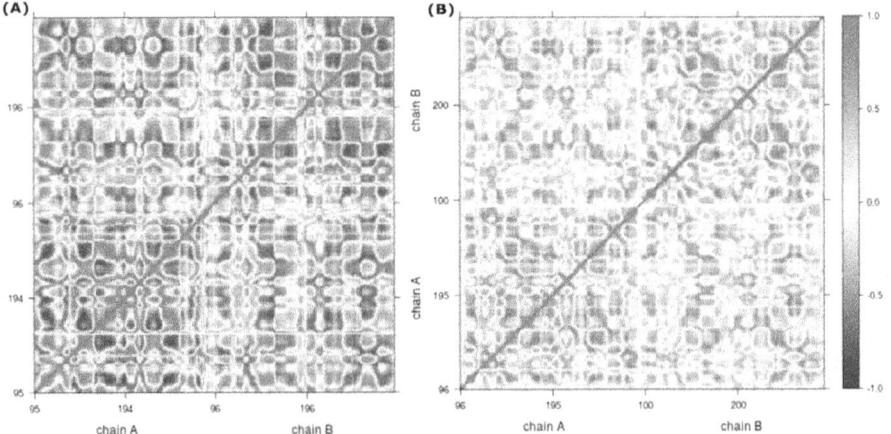

Figure 6: Dynamic cross correlation mapping. All atom correlation throughout 400ns MD simulation of p53-DBD as dimer in (A) DNA-A and (B) DNA-B complex.

Based on DCCM, the cut-off of 0.8-1.0 has been chosen to calculate the path for which residues are either positively or negatively correlated. K120, which is the DNA binding residue, was selected for calculating the allosteric path containing residues T155, C238 (corresponding to helix H1-loop L2 region), and T230 (corresponding to the loop consisting of residues from Y120 to T230) at the ends (**Figure 7**).

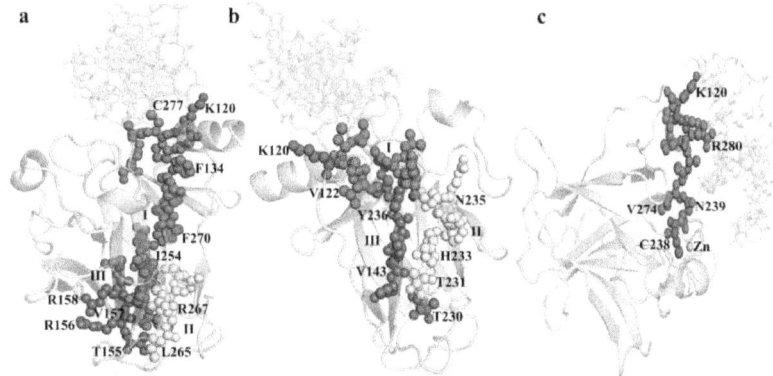

Figure 7 | Allosteric crosstalk. Communication path of p53-DBD-B between residues **a,** K120 and T155 **b,** K120 and T230 and **c,** K120 and Zn binding C238. Source and sink partners are colored red. Correlating residues along the path are represented in sphere and shown in magenta, marine and yellow for clarity

Chapter - II

Slow time scale motion in free and DNA-bound p53DBD: A comparison

Background:

In a cell, proteins functionally interact with other proteins forming a protein-protein interaction network, a characteristic of which is an organization around a few highly connected proteins called hubs.[73] Some of the hub proteins interact with tens to hundreds of proteins. The ability to interact with such diverse partners is created through many mechanisms, including post-translational chemical modifications. Even with such diversity-producing mechanisms, the repertoire of interaction surfaces may not be sufficiently broad to produce specific interactions with tens of partners. It has been proposed that besides other mechanisms, hub proteins have multiple conformational states near the ground state, and they access these otherwise invisible states to interact with different proteins.[74] Binding of ligands or chemical modifications may alter the ensemble of conformations, allowing selection of a specific set of interactions to take place, which is otherwise energetically unfavorable, thus creating a ligand/chemical modification specific subset of protein partners.[75] This proposed mechanism may be crucial for hub proteins to regulate specific pathways depending on the input received.

p53, a transcription factor and the master regulator of genomic integrity, plays crucial roles in a very large number of cellular functions.[76] It plays a dominant role in the process of carcinogenesis.[77] The participation of p53 in diverse cellular pathways involves interactions with hundreds of partner proteins, and thus, it has been termed a hub protein.[78] All its domains are involved in multiple protein-protein interactions, including the central DNA-binding domain (DBD), a small domain consisting of approximately 200 amino acids.[79] However, little is known about how such diverse interactions are accommodated within the limited surface repertoire of a small domain. One possibility is through post-translational chemical modifications, such as the acetylation of K120.[80] Another possibility is the presence of multiple conformational states which can be accessed to create a diverse repertoire of interfaces. We have investigated the latter possibility by Carr-Purcell-Meiboom-Gill (CPMG) NMR relaxation dispersion-based methods that probe molecular motions in the microseconds (μs) to milliseconds (ms) timescale. It is generally believed that conformational exchanges between the energetically close states occur on the slower μs-ms timescale.

Objective:

In this chapter, I have explored the conformational ensembles of the free and the DNA-bound p53-DBD through the chemical shift perturbation of backbone amides, and ^{15}N T_2 relaxation dispersion using the CPMG pulse sequence. I showed that the DNA-bound state, in contrast to the free-state, populates more than one state, interconverting on the millisecond timescale. I have discussed the implications of such observation for the protein-protein interactions of this hub protein.

Methods:

Sample preparation:

p53-DBD of ^{2}H (C-H protons), ^{15}N labeled p53 (residues 92-312), was expressed and purified as described previously. DNA sequences from IDT (Integrated DNA Technologies, USA) were annealed by heating to 95°C and then left for cooling at room temperature, annealing was verified by standard TOCSY and NOESY experiments. The DNA-p53 complex was formed by gradual mixing of small amounts of DNA (in 20 mM of Phosphate buffer, pH 6.9 containing 50 mM of KCl; stock concentration 1.5 mM) to p53 (stock concentration 320 μM) to avoid precipitation. An excess amount of 25% DNA was added to ensure complete titration of the protein for all the relaxation experiments.

NMR spectroscopy:

All NMR experiments for residue-specific backbone ^{15}N longitudinal (R_1) and rotating-frame relaxation ($R_{1\rho}$) rates were performed at 18°C on a Bruker Avance III 700 MHz (16.47 T field) spectrometer using a 5 mm QCI cryogenic probe equipped with z-axis gradients. The ^{1}H carrier was set at 4.7 ppm which is the frequency of the water resonance, while the ^{15}N carrier frequency was set to 118.5 ppm. These experiments were typically conducted with the pulse sequences with gradient and sensitivity-enhanced techniques by using flip-back and 3-9-19 binomial pulses for water suppression. Compensation pulses were applied before the recycle delay to ensure a constant radiofrequency (RF) load for the entire experiment, ensuring that there is a minimum sample heating effect amongst spectra employing a variable number of high-power RF pulses. ^{15}N quadrature detection was done with the echo-anti-echo method during $t1$ evolution. Free and the DNA-bound p53-DBD were assigned by three-dimensional HNCA, HNCACB experiments. The backbone amide ^{15}N spin-lattice relaxation (R_1), rotating frame relaxation ($R_{1\rho}$) dispersion experiments were performed following the pulse schemes developed by Lakomek et al.[81] For R_1 and $R_{1\rho}$ rate measurements, ^{15}N-^{1}H HSQC spectra were recorded with relaxation delays of 0, 480, 880, 160, 640, 320, 1200 ms and 5, 80, 1, 20, 40, 10, 120 ms, respectively. Carr-Purcell-Meiboom-Gill (CPMG) relaxation dispersion for backbone ^{15}N data was collected using a pulse sequence developed by Kay[82], with a total relaxation time (T_{relax}) of 40 ms. One control experiment without any CPMG relaxation delay (i.e. T_{relax} = 0) and two sets of triplicate measurements were acquired for error estimation. The number of ^{15}N CPMG π-pulses applied during the total relaxation time, T_{relax}, determined the CPMG π-pulse frequency (ν_{CPMG}) as follows:

$$\nu_{CPMG} = 1/2(2\tau_{cp} + t_{180,N})$$

Where $2\tau_{cp}$ is the spacing between two ^{15}N CPMG pulses and $t_{180,N}$ is the ^{15}N 180° pulse width used during CPMG relaxation delay. The effective transverse relaxation rates ($R_{2,eff} \pm \Delta R_{2,eff}$) for the backbone ^{15}N spins were extracted from the ^{15}N CPMG relaxation dispersion experiments following the equations:

$$R_{2,eff}(\nu_{CPMG}) = -1/T_{relax} \ln[I(\nu_{CPMG})/I_0]$$

$$\Delta R_{2,eff}(\nu_{CPMG}) = 1/T_{relax} \ln[\Delta I/I(\nu_{CPMG})]$$

where, $\Delta R_{2,eff}$ is the error in the measurement of $R_{2,eff}$, T_{relax} is the constant time relaxation period of 40 ms, ΔI is the root mean square error in $I(\nu_{CPMG})$, I_0 is the intensity of an amide peak corresponding to control spectrum ($T_{relax} = 0$), $I(\nu_{CPMG})$ is the intensity of an amide peak corresponding to a particular CPMG frequency, ΔI was obtained from two sets of triplicate measurements at high and low CPMG frequencies. The $R_{2,eff}$ values, obtained for each residue from 16.47 T external magnetic field, were plotted against ν_{CPMG} and fitted using the Catia[8] program to obtain simulated curves. Based on the results of this calculation, an initial identification of backbone amide ^{15}N spins subject to chemical exchange was performed as follows. For each residue, the simulated CPMG relaxation dispersion trajectories at 700 MHz external magnetic fields were used to calculate the corresponding exchange contributions. The chemical exchange contribution to ^{15}N R_2 i.e. R_{ex} was calculated from the difference in simulated $R_{2,eff}$ at the highest and lowest CPMG frequencies as follows:

$$R_{ex} = R_{2,eff}(\nu_{CPMG} = 25 Hz) - R_{2,eff}(\nu_{CPMG} = 1000 Hz) \quad (4)$$

All NMR spectra were processed with NMRPipe program[9]. Visualization and spectral assignments of p53 protein were done using Sparky. A Lorentzian-to-Gaussian multiplication window was applied to the FIDs prior to the Fourier transformation to process all the spectra. The peaks were fitted to a Gaussian line shape using nLinLS sub-routine in NMRPipe. The peak intensities were extracted and the trajectories of peak intensities were plotted against relaxation delays. Fitting the peak intensities to a single exponential function helped to extract the residue-specific relaxation rates for R_1 and $R_{1\rho}$. The transverse (R_2) relaxation rates were then calculated as a function of R_1, $R_{1\rho}$ rates as well as spin-lock field and ^{15}N frequency offset. The *r2r1_tm* program developed by Dr. Arthur G. Palmer (Columbia University) was used to estimate the rotational correlation time (τ_c). The initial estimation of τ_c was made from the R_2/R_1 ratio as input.

Results and Discussion:

To examine the dynamic character of the p53-DBD-DNA complex, we chose an oligonucleotide for which the protein-DNA co-complex crystal structure was known. Detailed knowledge of the structure would allow a more detailed interpretation of NMR data. The oligonucleotide duplex in the crystal structure (PDB id: 3KMD) was used as the p53 binding site. In this crystal structure, a 19-mer self-complementary oligonucleotide with one base overhang (5'-GGGCATGCCTAGGCATGCC-3') was co-crystallized with the tetramer of p53-DBD. This oligonucleotide, upon duplex formation, creates an 18 base pair double-stranded inverted repeat stretch with one base overhang. The p53-DBD is a monomer in the solution but tetramerizes in the presence of the above-mentioned DNA. To prevent tetramerization, which is likely to complicate NMR studies, we worked with a 10 base oligonucleotide, consisting of the 9 bp half-site with a C added to the 3' end to create a 10 base-paired duplex (a self-complementary oligonucleotide duplex with the sequence 5'-GGGCATGCCC-3').

We initially explored the chemical shift changes in the p53-DBD upon binding the DNA. Under these conditions, the DNA bound p53-DBD is in fast exchange with the free protein. **Figure 1a** shows the change in backbone amide chemical shift, $\Delta\delta_{amide}$, for a large majority of amide protons, obtained using the following equation:

$$\Delta\delta_{amide} = \sqrt{(\Delta\delta_{HN})^2 + (\Delta\delta_N/5)^2}$$

Where, $\Delta\delta_{HN}$ and $\Delta\delta_N$ denote ^1H and ^{15}N chemical shifts of the backbone amide, respectively.

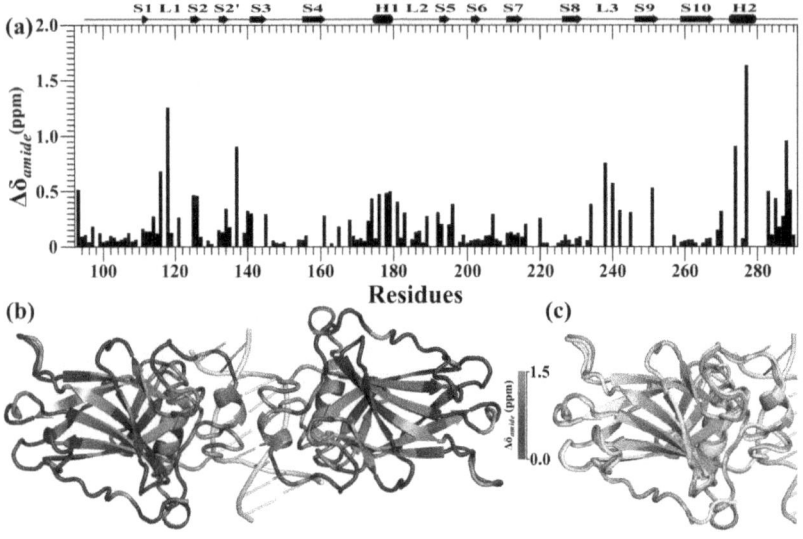

Figure 1. (a) **Change in amide chemical shift.** (b) p53 DNA-binding domain dimer in complex with DNA (pdb id: 3KMD). Only the half-site is shown as the half-site oligo was used in the solution experiments reported here. Missing residues are colored gray (c) Superposition of DNA-bound (cyan) and free p53-DBD (magenta, pdb id. 2OCJ).

At a DNA: protein molar ratio of 1:2, several amide protons show chemical shift changes above 0.5 ppm. When these residues were mapped on the structure of the DNA-protein complex (3KMD), they fall proximal to either the protein-DNA or the subunit-subunit interface (**Figure 1b**). It is likely that the chemical shift changes are the results of direct interaction with the DNA or proximity to the other subunit. The structural alignment of Chains A of the crystal structure of the free (PDB id: 2OCJ) and the DNA-bound complex (PDB id: 3KMD) shows (**Figure 1c**) that the backbones of the two structures align well with an overall RMSD of 0.54 Å. It may thus be tentatively concluded that the p53DBD binds to the DNA half-site, and the binding does not create major allosteric changes in the p53DBD.

In recent times, a significant hypothesis has emerged that native proteins exist in multiple interconverting conformations. A ligand may bind to only one of these conformations, pulling the equilibrium to a single conformer, a phenomenon known as the conformational selection. Multiple ligands may bind to different conformers. Thus, having a repertoire of conformations may allow a protein to interact with various partners, a requirement for a hub protein. To explore the possibility of the existence of conformational exchange in the p53DBD, we have studied the dynamics of this domain in the free and the DNA-bound state using NMR relaxation methods.

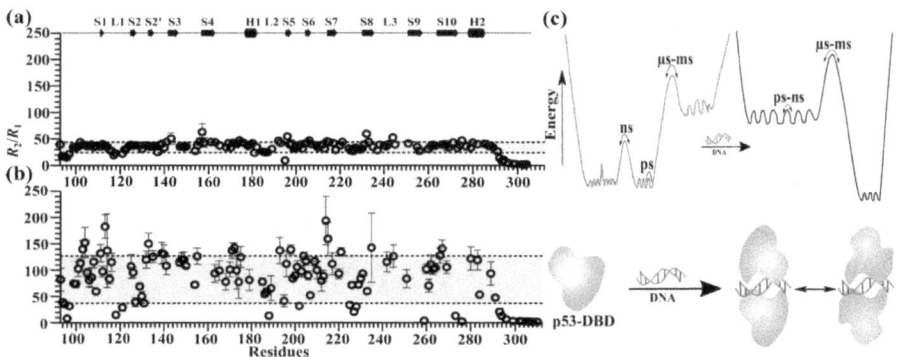

Figure 2. Fast time scale motion. R_2/R_1 values of (a) free p53-DBD and (b) DNA-bound p53-DBD. (c) Cartoon representation of energy landscape and conformational alterations to be more specific the effect of DNA binding.

Measurement of spin-lattice (R_1) and spin-spin (R_2) relaxation rates and their ratio (R_2/R_1) can give us a glimpse into dynamical characters of amino acid residues in the protein. The R_2/R_1 values of the free p53-DBD fall within a narrow range for most of the protein residues except those in the C-terminal region. This may indicate that the protein tumbles as a whole in the monomeric free-state with substantial segmental flexibility in the C-terminus. The DNA-bound p53-DBD, on the other hand, displays a much wider range of R_2/R_1 values, indicating significant differences in internal flexibility. The average of R_2/R_1 values is 34 ±10 (mean ± SD)

(**Figure 2a**) for the free DBD and 76±41 for that of the p53-DBD in complex with the DNA (**Figure 2b**). The free form has an estimated rotational correlation time (τ_c) of ~15 ns, which is indicative of a perdeuterated monomer, calculated from the R_2/R_1 ratio using the *r2r1_tm* program. The estimated τ_c of the p53-DBD in complex with DNA is ~27 ns, consistent with the formation of a dimer-DNA complex. In general, most of the residues in the DNA-bound state show higher R_2/R_1 values compared to their values in the free state, indicating a substantial increase in rigidity upon DNA-binding. However, some residues in the bound state, show very low R_2/R_1 values indicating enhanced flexibility (**Figure 2b**). The latter category of residues includes T119 and S121 belonging to the loop L1, residues V225, S227, and D228 belonging to the loop between S7 and S8 and residues R273 and A276.

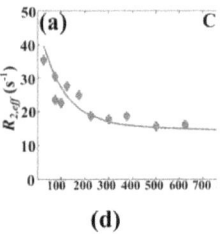

(d)

Figure 3. Slow time scale motion of p53DBD/DNA complex. Representative dispersion profile of ^{15}N backbone amides of p53-DBD complexed with DNA for residues (a) Zn binding C238 and (b) L289. (c) Indicates representative residue T150 that is not showing any kind of dispersion. The exchange rate (R_{ex}) has been mapped on the crystal structure where red color indicates residues with R_{ex}>5 s-1 and blue color represents residues with no dispersion (R_{ex}<3 s^{-1}). Missing residues are colored grey.

R_{ex} values were obtained from the difference of $R_{2,eff}$ values of the simulated trajectory at the highest and lowest CPMG frequencies, by fitting the data points as shown in the plot of $R_{2,eff}$ as a function of CPMG frequency (**Figure 3a-c**). R_{ex} values reflect the increase in the backbone dynamics of p53-DBD on slow timescales (**Figure 3a-c**). The slow timescale motion is very different in the p53-DBD/DNA complex compared to that in the free-state. The free form does not show significant relaxation dispersion with R_{ex} values close to zero for all residues, whereas in the DNA complex, residues corresponding to regions of dimerization interface (helix H1), DNA-binding surface (helix H2) show considerable chemical exchange. Remarkably, distant residues like T155 (terminal residue to sheet S4) and T230 (terminal residue to sheet S7) show significant conformational exchange. We also observe the dispersion for the Zn-binding residue C238, which undergoes the exchange process in µs-ms time scale. When highlighted on the 3KMD structure, residues that undergo slow exchange are scattered throughout the structure (**Figure 3d**).

For the DNA-binding domain, a small and relatively rigid domain, to show such promiscuous interactions, it may have to create diverse surface amino acid configurations. The R_{ex} values in the DNA-bound state suggest the domain samples different conformations while bound to a particular response element. In a previous molecular dynamics study, slow exchange in some distant residues in the DNA-bound state has been observed. The low chemical exchange was also deduced in selectively isotope-labeled protein by NMR as well. Many of the dynamic residues observed here are on the bottom outside surface of the full-length tetramer, making these residues accessible to partner proteins. Thus, multiple conformations of the DNA-bound tetramer may present an exposed repertoire of surface configuration, making them amenable to interaction with multiple partners. In the DNA-bound form, p53 can interact with several transcription factors and other classes of proteins while bound to Response Elements. As shown in Tuncbag et al.,[79] a large number of proteins interact with the DNA-binding domain and the interfaces for such protein-protein interactions are predicted to be different, but overlapping.

p53 stands at the cross-road of many cellular pathways and plays a crucial role in regulating these pathways.[83] It is by definition a hub protein. Its ability to present multiple surface architecture through visiting multiple conformations while bound to the response elements adds a new dimension to activating novel pathways upon DNA-binding.[83,84] We speculate that such conformational diversity may be present in other transcription factors as well in their DNA-bound state.

Chapter -III

Electrostatic modulation in molecular recognition by p53

Background:

In this chapter I have addressed a very fundamental question, the role of non-bonded electrostatics behind the allosteric response in molecular recognition of the DNA binding domain of p53 (p53DBD). I have selected atomic structures of p53DBD in complex with either DNA or a repressor protein iASPP and used MD simulation approach for that purpose. The DNA binding domain of p53 (p53DBD) consists of a β-sandwich scaffold that supports the loop–sheet helix (LSH) motif which interacts with the major groove of RE where the L3 loop connects minor groove along with the DNA backbone.[17] The LSH includes DNA-binding R280 from the H2 helix and K120 from the L1 loop which involves target selection. On the other hand, iASPP belongs to the family of ASPP (apoptosis stimulating protein of p53) and acts as a repressor of p53 by segregating the L1 loop of p53.[85] Notably, p53DBD binds to both the factors with similar affinities (binding affinities for DNA and iASPP binding are 20±3 nM and 26.4±1.7 nM respectively).[86,87]

Backbone overlay of crystal structures of the two complexes (with DNA and iASPP) revealed virtually no conformational changes in p53DBD except the L1 loop, despite the fact that distal residue mutation (like R213) in p53DBD can alter its binding affinity indicating that dynamic allostery plays a pivotal role. A recent study reported that dynamic allostery in a protein is not resulted from entropic effect alone and can not be captured sometimes only by structure and dynamics, as traditionally believed, modulation in internal electrostatic energy profile also contributes significantly in the process.[88]

Objective:

In this chapter, my aim was to understand the communication path for allosteric responses and nonbonded energy contributions for molecular recognition in these complexes. To this end, MD simulation studies were performed with p53DBD-DNA and p53DBD-iASPP complexes followed by meticulous analysis of residue-wise non-bonded contribution (individually with

DNA or iASPP) and pairwise interaction energies of p53DBD. In line with the previous finding[88], the electrostatic energy revealed an evolutionarily conserved allosteric crosstalk (information of which was not obtained from structure or dynamics) and reorganization of path connecting the binding- to allosteric sites. Perturbations of specific pair-wise electrostatic interactions occur due to distance population shift in the two complexes of p53DBD.

Materials and Methods:

MOLECULAR DYNAMICS

The DNA and iASPP bound p53DBD crystal structures (PDB ID: 3KMD (chain C was extracted to construct monomer-DNA complex, residues 92-291) and 6RZ3, residues 92-291, respectively) were equilibrated for 1 ns with capping the C and N termini of both by N-methyl amide and acetyl groups. All MD simulations were performed on GROMACS 5.1.2 software[69] using *Amber99SB-Ildn* force field[68] and TIP3P water model[71] with a box size of 1 nm. The protonation states for the titratable residues were determined using MCCE (multi-conformation continuum electrostatics) method[89] and also from PROPKA Web server[90] with respect to pH 7.4. Parameters for the Zn ion were used based on the forcefield. The systems were neutralized by adding 150 mM NaCl by substituting appropriate numbers of solvent molecules to mimic experimental salt condition. The structures were energy minimized followed by two-step equilibration, namely NVT equilibration followed by NPT equilibration. Temperature was controlled through velocity rescaling[91] at 310 K with a time constant of 0.1 ps, and pressure was controlled using Parrinello–Rahman barostat[92] at 1 bar. The particle mesh Ewald algorithm was applied to calculate long-range electrostatic interactions.[93] The cutoff for short-range electrostatics and van der Waals' interaction was 1.2 nm. MD simulations of 1.0 μs for each complexes were performed and frames were recorded at every 2 ps.[94] Stabilization and convergence of simulations in both the complexes were ensured by Root Mean Square Deviation (RMSD).

Differential contact map and Dynamic cross correlation matrix (DCCM)

Last frame from the final MD simulation for both the complexes were extracted using a tool provided by Gromacs. The contact was defined between any two atoms of two residues by specifying their distance within 4.5 Å.[95] Differential contact map was generated from two same dimension contact matrices (one for p53DBD-DNA and other for p53DBD-iASPP complexes, only p53DBD was considered here).

Cross-correlation maps are used to identify the regions that move in or out of phase during the simulations.[72] The elements of the matrix (C_{ij}) were obtained from their position vector (r) as shown in Eq. 1:

$$C_{ij} = \frac{\langle (r_i - \langle r_i \rangle)(r_j - \langle r_j \rangle) \rangle}{\sqrt{(\langle r_i^2 \rangle - \langle r_i \rangle^2)(\langle r_j^2 \rangle - \langle r_j \rangle^2)}}$$

Where i and j correspond to any two atoms, residues, or domains; r_i and r_j are position vectors of i and j; and the angle brackets denote an ensemble average. Interatomic cross-correlation fluctuations between any two pairs of atoms (or residues) can be calculated by using this expression and can be represented graphically by the DCCM. The value of C_{ij} can vary from -1 (completely anti-correlated motion) to +1 (completely correlated motion).

Order parameter (S^2)

Backbone N-H vectors were selected to calculate S^2 over the period of trajectory, which represent dynamicity of protein with the value 1 indicates complete rigidity and towards 0 represents enhanced dynamicity.

$$S^2 = \frac{1}{2} \langle 3 \sum_{i=1}^{3} \sum_{j=1}^{3} \langle \mu_i \mu_j \rangle^2 - 1 \rangle$$

in which μ1, μ2, and μ3 are the x, y, and z components of the relevant bond vector scaled to unit magnitude, μ, respectively.[96] Angular brackets indicate averaging over the snapshots.

Energy perturbation

The residue wise nonbonded interaction energy between p53 with its two binding substrate (DNA and iASPP) was described as:

$$\Delta E^{p53-substrate}_{nonbonded} = \Delta E^{p53-substrate}_{electrostatic} + \Delta E^{p53-substrate}_{VDW}$$

The nonbonded interactions ($\Delta E_{nonbonded}$) include both electrostatic ($\Delta E_{electrostatic}$) and van der Waals (ΔE_{VDW}) interactions and were modeled using a Coulomb and Lennard-Jones (LJ) potential function, respectively. A cutoff of 2 nm was applied for computing interaction energy with water molecules. The contributions due to LJ and electrostatic (Coulomb) nonbonded interactions to $\Delta E_{nonbonded}$ were calculated separately, but the LJ terms were found to be numerically much smaller than the respective electrostatic ones, so we have focused on the electrostatic interactions while calculating the perturbation in pair-wise interactions $\Delta E_{i\text{-}j}$.

$$\Delta E_{i-j} = \Delta E^{electrostatic}_{i-j} + \Delta E^{VDW}_{i-j} \approx \Delta E^{electrostatic}_{i-j}$$

The interaction energy between two residues i and j is the sum of the non-bonded interaction energies already defined in a force-field where

$$\Delta E^{electrostatic}_{i-j} = \varsigma \frac{q_i q_j}{\varepsilon_r r_{ij}}, \varsigma = \frac{1}{4\Pi\varepsilon_0} = 138.935485$$

$$\Delta E^{VDW}_{i-j} = 4\varepsilon_{ij}((\frac{\sigma_{ij}}{r_{ij}})^{12} - (\frac{\sigma_{ij}}{r_{ij}})^{6}), \sigma_{ij} = \frac{1}{2}(\sigma_{ii} + \sigma_{jj}), \varepsilon_{ij} = (\varepsilon_{ii}\varepsilon_{jj})^{\frac{1}{2}}$$

Energy network, construction of energy Hubs and shortest path

Energy networks are built by considering the amino-acid residues as nodes. A weighted edge is made between any pair of residues *i* and *j* by considering the interaction energy (Eq. 4) as the weight. Energy-Hubs are defined as nodes that have a higher degree or connectivity in the network. Note that for better comparison we have considered the same Hubs in both the complexes.

Betweenness-Centrality was computed using the following equation:

$$BC(v) = \frac{2}{(n-1)(n-2)} \sum_{i \neq v \neq j \in E} \frac{\sigma_{ij}(v)}{\sigma_{ij}}$$

Where BC(v) is betweenness-centrality of residue v. n is the number of residues within a network, $\sigma_{ij}(v)$ is the number of shortest paths between residue i and j that pass through residue v and σ_{ij} is the total number of shortest paths from i to j.

Results and discussion

Overall structure and dynamicity of p53DBD in complex with DNA or iASPP:

Structural difference restricted only to loop regions (e.g. loop L2, L3, and loops connecting beta sheets S4-S3, S6-S7, S7-S8 and S9-S10) in p53DBD was observed when the backbone traces of the simulated crystal structures (i.e. final conformations of the simulations) of its complexes with DNA and iASPP were overlaid (**Figure 1A**).

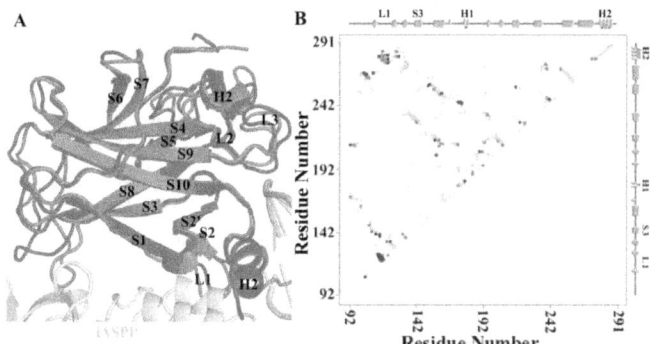

Figure 1. (**A**) Superposition of final simulated structure of p53DBD in the DNA bound state (PDB ID: 3KMD, colored in red) and iASPP bound state (PDB ID: 6RZ3, colored in blue). DNA and iASPP are colored in salmon and palecyan respectively. (**B**) Differential contact map between DNA and iASPP bound simulated structures. Contacts exclusively present in DNA and iASPP bound states are shown in red and blue respectively where the common contacts are colored gray. Most of the differential contacts appear in binding regions to respective binding partners (here DNA and iASPP).

We then focused on the p53DBD side-chain reorganizations, occurring through rotameric alteration dynamics, in these two complexes. Residue pair-wise contact map is a widely used tool for identifying differences in side chain conformations.[97] It has been postulated that, for allosteric involvement, contacts of neighboring residues are more likely coupled compared to the distal ones[98], and different contact-based frameworks has been proposed to evaluate structural basis for the transmission of information.[99] Following similar methodology, the differential contact matrix was constructed (**Figure 1B**) based on the final state of simulated structures of p53DBD-DNA and p53DBD-iASPP complexes to find differences in the side-chain contacts in p53DBD. The contacts for p53DBD-DNA and p53DBD-iASPP were mapped in red and blue, respectively. It is seen that most of the pair-wise contacts are common (grey regions). However, few contacts are exclusively present in either of the complexes. Interestingly, these complex-specific contacts occur in the region of interactions with the binding partners. Nevertheless, the side-chain contact map reflects minor structural rearrangements in p53DBD upon DNA/repressor binding.

Apparently, dynamicity plays a crucial role behind the energy modulation in the two complexes. We have calculated residue wise root mean square fluctuations (RMSF) based on Cα atoms and Order Parameter (S^2) of N-H vectors with the anticipation that fluctuations of Cα atoms and N-H vectors would provide deeper insight on backbone dynamicity. Overall fluctuations with respect to Cα increases due to repressor binding compared to DNA-binding (**Figure 2A**). Noticeable changes were observed in loop regions e.g. loop between beta sheets S3 and S4; residue number V147-T155, beta sheets S7 and S8; residue number Y220-C229 and sheet S9 and S10; residue number D259-N263. Interestingly however, the loop L1 (residues F113 to C124), having both DNA-binding (K120) and iASPP-binding (H115) residues, shows decrement in Cα fluctuations in repressor-binding as compared to DNA-binding (**Figure 2A**) indicating a role of L1 dynamicity too behind the loss of p53DBD activity upon complex formation with iASPP. On the other hand, N-H bond fluctuations calculated from Order Parameter (S^2) showed almost similar overall backbone dynamicity of p53DBD in both the complexes except loop L3 that contains DNA-binding residue R248 and Zn-binding residues C238 and C242. The dynamic regions from S^2 successfully capture those of free p53DBD derived from NMR.[100] Thus, in contrast to the minute changes in overall N-H fluctuations Cα dynamics show pronounced alterations.

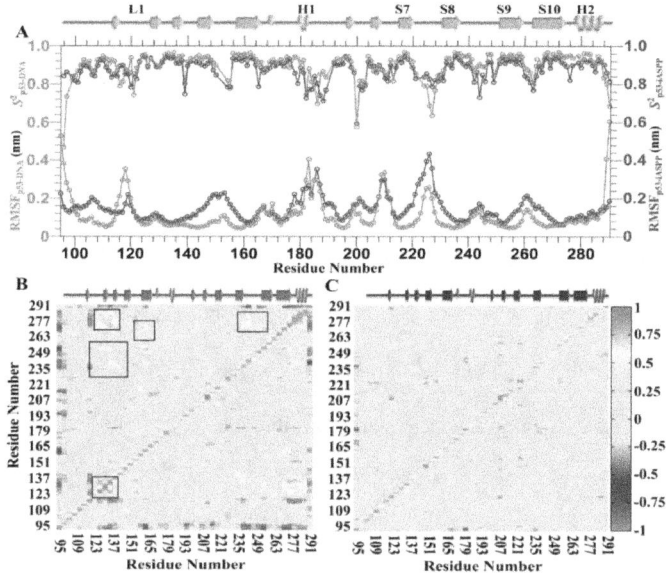

Figure 2. (**A**) Comparison of Backbone dynamicity of p53DBD bound individually with DNA (red) and iASPP (blue), based on residue wise RMSF and Order Parameter (S^2). Information of S^2 for Proline residues are missing due to their lack of N-H bonds. Dynamic cross correlation (strong: $|C_{ij}| = 1.0–0.7$; moderate: $|C_{ij}| = 0.7–0.5$; and

weak: $|C_{ij}| = 0.3–0.5$) within residues of p53DBD are represented in the form of matrix in (**B**) with DNA bound state and (**C**) with iASPP bound state. Differential areas in DNA bound state are indicated by box and actually establishing correlation between DNA and Zn binding regions, which are missing in iASPP bound state.

In recent studies Dynamic Cross Correlation Matrix (DCCM, C_{ij}) based approach has gained much attention for determining dynamic allostery in proteins through monitoring correlated motions among residues.[101] Correlated and anti-correlated motions score between 1 and -1 (strong: $|C_{ij}| = 1.0–0.7$; moderate: $|C_{ij}| = 0.7–0.5$; and weak: $|C_{ij}| = 0.3– 0.5$). We have calculated DCCM of p53DBD in both the complexes to predict the presence of any distal correlations. Interestingly, DNA-binding region of p53DBD containing residues K120, R248, R273, C277, R280 as well as Zn-binding residues C238 and C242 appears to have moderate correlation in presence of DNA which is completely missing in the complex with iASPP (**Figure 2B** and **2C**) suggesting the correlated motions of the above mentioned residues in DNA-binding state is significant as reported earlier compared to the same in repressor-binding state.[102,103] In agreement with this conclusion, further dynamic correlations between L1 and helix H2 to Zn-binding loop L2 appeared to be crucial in DNA-binding state.

Although differential alteration in the overall dynamicity of p53DBD is observed in two complexes, the mechanism how the distal residues contribute in molecular recognition is still not clear. So, we further explored the intra-protein interaction energy network to understand the dynamics governed by intrinsic electrostatic contributions.

Contributions of nonbonded interactions in p53DBD complexes with DNA and iASPP:

It is clear that structure and dynamics of p53DBD could not explain functional contribution of the distal residues, reported earlier.[104] Hence, we step forward to evaluate more fundamental electrostatic and van der Waals interaction energies. It has been well established that protein undergoes a drastic perturbation in energy at its binding site upon complex formation which propagates through the intra-protein network to the allosteric sites. Following MD simulation, we have computed the alteration in the residue-wise nonbonded interaction energy in terms of the electrostatic ($\Delta E_{electrostatic}^{p53-substrate}$) and van der Waals' ($\Delta E_{VDW}^{p53-substrate}$) of p53DBD complexes with DNA and the repressor (**Figure 3A** and **3B**) based on the procedure described earlier.[105]

A global diminution of residue-wise electrostatic energy in p53DBD is observed when bound to iASPP as compared to its DNA-bound state. Remarkable variations in the electrostatic energy ($\Delta E_{electrostatic} = \Delta E_{electrostatic}^{p53-DNA} - \Delta E_{electrostatic}^{p53-iASPP}$) (up to ~150 kcal/mol) was observed between p53DBD-DNA and p53DBD-iASPP interactions, although the contributing residues remain the same in both (**Figure 3A**) suggesting that a common electrostatic framework has been used by p53DBD while complexing with its partner, irrespective of its mode of action. On the other hand, the van der Waals' interaction energy ($\Delta E_{VDW} = \Delta E_{VDW}^{p53-DNA} - \Delta E_{VDW}^{p53-iASPP}$) profile shows a modest range of variation up to ~6 kcal/mol (**Figure 3B**). Evidently, electrostatic interaction energy is the predominant factor in nonbonded interaction energy (**Table 1-4**).

Table 1. Residue wise electrostatic contributions of p53DBD towards iASPP in kcal/mol

Residues	$\Delta E_{electro}$	± Error	Residues	$\Delta E_{electro}$	± Error	Residues	$\Delta E_{electro}$	± Error	Residues	$\Delta E_{electro}$	± Error
92	0.717	0.093	142	0.849	0.560	192	0.715	0.331	242	0.311	0.310
93	-0.377	0.130	143	-0.992	0.106	193	0.658	0.229	243	0.44	0.350
94	0.224	0.373	144	-4.308	2.824	194	0.305	0.140	244	-0.042	0.305
95	0.221	0.261	145	0.804	0.204	195	-0.979	0.121	245	-0.174	0.300
96	0.047	0.185	146	-1.178	0.269	196	-54.05	1.017	246	0.032	0.228
97	-0.231	0.155	147	0.745	0.236	197	-0.997	0.093	247	0.119	0.220
98	0.368	0.128	148	73.964	10.121	198	67.839	2.006	248	-59.034	4.230
99	0.538	0.301	149	0.26	0.540	199	0.127	0.595	249	-56.211	1.365
100	1.15	1.083	150	0.162	0.265	200	-1.572	0.313	250	-1.285	0.160
101	-70.56	5.906	151	-0.149	0.230	201	-0.445	0.097	251	1.133	0.099
102	-0.78	0.530	152	0.618	0.063	202	-54.16	2.925	252	-1.064	0.101
103	-0.219	0.470	153	0.007	0.198	203	-0.849	0.060	253	0.551	0.149
104	-1.532	1.235	154	-0.226	0.101	204	51.217	1.294	254	-0.524	0.107
105	1.596	0.191	155	-0.008	0.220	205	-0.283	0.076	255	0.259	0.092
106	0.816	0.458	156	-53.79	1.499	206	0.489	0.046	256	-0.092	0.263
107	0.36	0.274	157	-0.681	0.110	207	48.473	1.579	257	-0.093	0.158
108	0.702	0.426	158	-55.48	1.829	208	52.767	3.638	258	57.752	2.037
109	0.622	0.432	159	-0.831	0.060	209	-47.68	3.915	259	54.765	1.771
110	-90.46	7.178	160	0.84	0.174	210	-0.791	0.666	260	-0.365	0.165
111	1.199	0.299	161	-0.828	0.042	211	-0.108	0.170	261	-0.36	0.215
112	-1.542	0.363	162	0.823	0.035	212	-0.041	0.251	262	0.065	0.162
113	1.536	0.381	163	-0.021	0.398	213	-55.3	1.454	263	0	0.472
114	-2.625	0.558	164	-75.52	2.110	214	1.47	0.166	264	-0.305	0.153
115	-6.48	3.368	165	-0.996	0.693	215	-0.745	0.115	265	0.637	0.125
116	1.571	1.034	166	-0.455	0.421	216	0.521	0.105	266	-0.971	0.243
117	-0.34	0.396	167	-0.407	0.455	217	-0.378	0.093	267	-64.817	2.982
118	1.847	1.125	168	0.021	0.692	218	0.137	0.099	268	-0.645	0.620
119	0.57	1.004	169	-0.08	0.355	219	0.957	0.102	269	1.304	0.425
120	-74.64	7.463	170	-0.08	0.175	220	-1.363	0.461	270	-1.271	0.131
121	0.321	1.264	171	53.245	1.112	221	63.234	2.782	271	80.701	1.915
122	-1.98	0.413	172	-0.114	0.052	222	-0.495	0.205	272	-0.465	0.165
123	-0.449	0.667	173	-0.328	0.120	223	-1.763	0.438	273	-75.415	2.032
124	0.937	0.756	174	-48.29	0.789	224	68.486	4.392	274	-0.302	0.202
125	-2.825	0.641	175	-53.2	1.175	225	1.019	0.645	275	0.228	0.614
126	1.991	0.591	176	0.139	0.247	226	1.121	1.021	276	0.182	0.378
127	-3.125	0.385	177	-0.039	0.116	227	-2.697	1.467	277	0.16	0.595
128	-3.492	0.726	178	-0.557	0.429	228	86.54	8.769	278	1.015	0.272
129	-3.366	1.143	179	-0.298	0.218	229	0.983	0.850	279	0.714	1.629
130	-1.973	0.188	180	46.428	1.017	230	1.45	0.500	280	-80.02	3.913
131	-3.921	1.558	181	-43.26	1.556	231	-0.226	1.021	281	80.13	2.217
132	-80.16	1.653	182	-0.201	0.344	232	1.549	0.312	282	-131.82	3.940
133	-1.985	0.238	183	-0.24	0.237	233	-1.755	1.072	283	-105.08	10.500
134	1.195	0.191	184	50.61	2.860	234	1.086	0.462	284	1.385	0.720
135	-0.732	0.318	185	-0.061	0.185	235	-1.708	0.098	285	84.569	2.185
136	0.56	0.735	186	52.01	1.161	236	0.678	0.110	286	111.03	2.533
137	0.383	0.137	187	-0.452	0.180	237	0.051	0.065	287	106.79	10.603
138	-0.438	0.118	188	-0.47	0.233	238	0.511	0.075	288	0.492	1.011
139	-65.8	1.935	189	-0.246	0.247	239	-0.89	0.854	289	1.257	1.274
140	1.024	0.268	190	0.878	0.050	240	-0.274	0.304	290	-118.57	6.350
141	-0.996	0.148	191	0.702	0.094	241	-0.401	0.468	291	3.031	9.576

Table 2. Residue wise van der Waals' contributions of p53DBD towards iASPP in kcal/mol

Residues	ΔE_{VDW}	± Error	Residues	ΔE_{VDW}	± Error	Residues	ΔE_{VDW}	± Error	Residues	ΔE_{VDW}	± Error
92	-0.001	0.000	142	-0.241	0.082	192	-0.001	0.000	242	-0.004	0.001
93	-0.001	0.000	143	-0.109	0.034	193	-0.003	0.000	243	-0.002	0.000
94	-0.001	0.000	144	-1.559	0.834	194	-0.005	0.001	244	-0.001	0.000
95	-0.001	0.000	145	-0.092	0.027	195	-0.008	0.001	245	-0.001	0.000
96	-0.001	0.000	146	-1.918	0.758	196	-0.007	0.001	246	-0.006	0.001
97	-0.003	0.001	147	-0.134	0.054	197	-0.008	0.001	247	-0.003	0.000
98	-0.004	0.001	148	0.568	1.209	198	-0.016	0.003	248	-0.007	0.002
99	-0.006	0.002	149	-0.048	0.020	199	-0.005	0.001	249	-0.006	0.001
100	-0.018	0.005	150	-0.02	0.006	200	-0.006	0.002	250	-0.01	0.002
101	-0.037	0.026	151	-0.013	0.004	201	-0.003	0.001	251	-0.014	0.002
102	-0.079	0.045	152	-0.005	0.001	202	-0.004	0.001	252	-0.02	0.005
103	-0.055	0.026	153	-0.003	0.001	203	-0.003	0.000	253	-0.018	0.003
104	-0.423	0.370	154	-0.001	0.000	204	-0.002	0.000	254	-0.015	0.003
105	-0.038	0.025	155	-0.005	0.001	205	-0.003	0.000	255	-0.026	0.007
106	-0.038	0.023	156	-0.006	0.001	206	-0.002	0.000	256	-0.011	0.003
107	-0.057	0.026	157	-0.011	0.002	207	-0.001	0.000	257	-0.017	0.004
108	-0.114	0.074	158	-0.008	0.001	208	-0.002	0.001	258	-0.006	0.001
109	-0.097	0.043	159	-0.005	0.001	209	-0.002	0.001	259	-0.003	0.001
110	-1.578	1.312	160	-0.007	0.001	210	-0.001	0.001	260	-0.001	0.000
111	-0.225	0.086	161	-0.004	0.001	211	-0.002	0.001	261	-0.001	0.000
112	-0.307	0.120	162	-0.008	0.001	212	-0.001	0.000	262	-0.001	0.000
113	-1.449	0.515	163	-0.007	0.001	213	-0.003	0.000	263	-0.004	0.001
114	-5.522	2.087	164	-0.021	0.004	214	-0.002	0.000	264	-0.009	0.003
115	-9.32	2.349	165	-0.007	0.001	215	-0.002	0.000	265	-0.013	0.005
116	-1.617	0.832	166	-0.004	0.001	216	-0.005	0.001	266	-0.01	0.004
117	-1.362	0.649	167	-0.003	0.000	217	-0.004	0.001	267	-0.031	0.012
118	-2.949	0.781	168	-0.004	0.000	218	-0.006	0.001	268	-0.072	0.030
119	-4.593	1.371	169	-0.005	0.001	219	-0.005	0.001	269	-0.037	0.010
120	-2.498	0.755	170	-0.002	0.000	220	-0.023	0.006	270	-0.081	0.017
121	-1.654	0.753	171	-0.002	0.000	221	-0.012	0.003	271	-0.054	0.010
122	-3.742	1.548	172	-0.002	0.000	222	-0.015	0.004	272	-0.031	0.005
123	-0.252	0.080	173	-0.003	0.000	223	-0.045	0.016	273	-0.056	0.007
124	-0.395	0.144	174	-0.002	0.000	224	-0.034	0.015	274	-0.019	0.003
125	-1.262	0.363	175	-0.003	0.000	225	-0.037	0.029	275	-0.036	0.007
126	-1.834	0.593	176	-0.001	0.000	226	-0.092	0.090	276	-0.027	0.005
127	-2.077	0.623	177	-0.001	0.000	227	-0.302	0.351	277	-0.138	0.034
128	-7.497	1.839	178	-0.001	0.000	228	-0.446	0.206	278	-0.286	0.094
129	-2.142	1.071	179	-0.002	0.000	229	-0.501	0.241	279	-1.116	0.814
130	-0.791	0.200	180	-0.001	0.000	230	-0.072	0.027	280	-1.297	0.648
131	-0.338	0.165	181	-0.001	0.000	231	-0.177	0.099	281	-0.18	0.040
132	-0.197	0.035	182	-0.001	0.000	232	-0.04	0.011	282	-2.545	1.129
133	-0.131	0.025	183	-0.001	0.000	233	-0.066	0.021	283	-5.702	1.377
134	-0.256	0.041	184	-0.001	0.001	234	-0.032	0.007	284	-0.265	0.083
135	-0.054	0.011	185	-0.001	0.000	235	-0.013	0.003	285	-0.242	0.021
136	-0.064	0.013	186	-0.002	0.000	236	-0.024	0.004	286	-3.834	1.423
137	-0.013	0.001	187	-0.001	0.000	237	-0.006	0.001	287	-1.165	0.633
138	-0.008	0.001	188	-0.002	0.000	238	-0.005	0.000	288	-0.289	0.045
139	-0.039	0.010	189	-0.001	0.000	239	-0.008	0.001	289	-2.503	1.040
140	-0.067	0.021	190	-0.001	0.000	240	-0.008	0.001	290	-10.719	2.058
141	-0.06	0.016	191	-0.001	0.000	241	-0.006	0.002	291	-3.214	3.477

Table 3. Residue wise electrostatic contributions of p53DBD towards DNA in kcal/mol

Residues	$\Delta E_{electro}$	± Error	Residues	$\Delta E_{electro}$	± Error	Residues	$\Delta E_{electro}$	± Error	Residues	$\Delta E_{electro}$	± Error
92	-92.83	1.552	142	1.6805	0.198	192	1.7464	1.106	242	-4.189	2.537
93	-0.422	0.437	143	-0.361	0.203	193	3.0279	0.605	243	-4.394	2.490
94	0.4295	0.476	144	0.7721	0.628	194	1.2645	0.370	244	-2.5483	0.512
95	1.6552	0.845	145	-0.204	0.132	195	-0.888	0.202	245	-2.2898	0.910
96	-0.242	0.995	146	-0.155	0.565	196	-93.15	3.727	246	-2.7429	1.054
97	0.4043	0.942	147	0.13	0.070	197	0.2398	0.254	247	0.1412	2.600
98	0.2831	0.733	148	60.779	0.825	198	94.299	1.834	248	-224.54	7.998
99	-0.217	0.617	149	0.7312	0.214	199	-0.686	0.247	249	-127.04	5.242
100	0.305	1.329	150	-0.289	0.183	200	-0.195	0.214	250	-1.9581	0.525
101	-68.93	1.713	151	-0.434	0.020	201	0.1214	0.333	251	1.1381	0.520
102	-0.692	0.487	152	0.9938	0.065	202	-61.78	1.368	252	0.9529	0.349
103	0.6026	0.193	153	0.039	0.392	203	-0.918	0.228	253	0.7412	0.399
104	-1.098	0.414	154	0.2314	0.137	204	67.112	1.931	254	0.6048	0.311
105	0.2081	0.117	155	0.1612	0.160	205	-0.486	0.179	255	0.02	0.156
106	-0.181	0.120	156	-64.4	1.982	206	1.2364	0.188	256	1.425	0.119
107	-0.095	0.157	157	-0.293	0.111	207	71.781	4.375	257	0.1845	0.044
108	0.3143	0.124	158	-72.24	1.668	208	73.231	2.025	258	67.774	1.638
109	-0.051	0.121	159	-0.75	0.093	209	-65.76	1.568	259	57.48	1.231
110	-67.95	1.055	160	0.0936	0.814	210	-0.08	0.937	260	0.3245	0.363
111	-1.079	0.192	161	-1.806	0.242	211	0.436	0.367	261	0.1017	0.415
112	0.0198	0.229	162	1.2452	0.239	212	1.4495	0.540	262	0.2731	0.266
113	-1.459	0.382	163	-1.716	0.272	213	-89.76	1.780	263	0.5376	0.257
114	1.3712	0.375	164	-117.4	3.720	214	1.5686	1.337	264	-0.9338	0.132
115	-0.148	0.625	165	-1.408	1.702	215	-0.725	0.550	265	-0.4364	0.109
116	-0.71	1.558	166	-0.011	0.438	216	0.1531	0.158	266	-0.1212	0.049
117	1.3255	1.019	167	-1.195	3.064	217	0.3843	0.180	267	-73.25	0.688
118	1.3879	2.424	168	-2.672	1.040	218	0.1936	0.086	268	-0.2129	1.137
119	2.524	1.575	169	-0.742	0.326	219	1.1752	0.134	269	-1.5405	0.755
120	-164.3	34.230	170	0.0467	0.619	220	-0.186	0.066	270	-0.7295	0.161
121	-4.558	1.480	171	112.37	3.439	221	65.443	0.549	271	123.53	2.891
122	4.5052	0.786	172	1.9507	0.337	222	0.4905	0.158	272	0.4569	0.329
123	2.2264	0.558	173	-2.56	0.252	223	-1.014	0.162	273	-212.85	7.365
124	-1.046	1.463	174	-102.2	3.708	224	61.342	3.773	274	5.2221	0.386
125	0.9214	0.403	175	-113.6	4.131	225	0.7748	0.304	275	-13.61	1.349
126	-0.231	0.451	176	-4.238	1.328	226	0.5455	0.248	276	-10.583	2.376
127	-1.026	0.705	177	-2.866	0.338	227	-0.283	0.780	277	-1.3736	1.972
128	-0.171	0.376	178	-6.825	0.590	228	63.431	1.413	278	0.4869	0.432
129	-0.949	0.223	179	-2.335	2.105	229	0.1036	0.415	279	-4.1426	2.034
130	-0.384	0.223	180	103.53	1.529	230	0.3745	0.198	280	-231.46	6.072
131	0.5964	0.642	181	-104.1	2.451	231	-0.478	0.093	281	202	3.380
132	-144.1	4.311	182	-0.697	0.852	232	0.7831	0.171	282	-119.51	1.280
133	2.5071	0.575	183	1.534	2.112	233	0.2388	1.241	283	-156.8	11.124
134	-3.404	0.513	184	103.66	4.833	234	0.7214	0.185	284	-2.5755	3.218
135	4.1981	1.083	185	0.2067	0.748	235	-3.535	0.924	285	151.49	9.389
136	-9.02	1.718	186	86.274	2.236	236	1.1588	0.215	286	117.88	2.816
137	-1.5	0.531	187	-1.233	0.307	237	1.22	0.405	287	131.11	9.617
138	-1.187	0.495	188	-0.636	0.919	238	-3.045	1.073	288	-3.9457	3.468
139	-129.2	6.529	189	0.6076	0.740	239	-10.61	5.797	289	-1.6505	0.513
140	2.5786	0.279	190	1.7448	0.251	240	-2.665	0.670	290	-129.7	36.094
141	0.4836	0.351	191	2.1445	0.257	241	-7.333	3.552			

Table 4. Residue wise van der Waals' contributions of p53DBD towards DNA in kcal/mol

Residues	ΔE$_{VDW}$	± Error	Residues	ΔE$_{VDW}$	± Error	Residues	ΔE$_{VDW}$	± Error	Residues	ΔE$_{VDW}$	± Error
92	-0.004	-0.001	142	-0.007	-0.002	192	-0.006	-0.001	242	-0.424	-0.101
93	-0.003	-0.001	143	-0.004	-0.001	193	-0.007	-0.002	243	-1.293	-0.308
94	-0.001	0.000	144	-0.002	0.000	194	-0.024	-0.006	244	-0.05	-0.012
95	-0.001	0.000	145	-0.001	0.000	195	-0.009	-0.002	245	-0.032	-0.008
96	-0.001	0.000	146	-0.001	0.000	196	-0.01	-0.002	246	-0.113	-0.027
97	-0.002	0.000	147	0	0.000	197	-0.003	-0.001	247	-0.239	-0.057
98	-0.001	0.000	148	0	0.000	198	-0.006	-0.001	248	-5.022	-1.196
99	-0.001	0.000	149	0	0.000	199	-0.001	0.000	249	-0.15	-0.036
100	-0.003	-0.001	150	0	0.000	200	-0.001	0.000	250	-0.085	-0.020
101	-0.001	0.000	151	0	0.000	201	-0.001	0.000	251	-0.041	-0.010
102	-0.001	0.000	152	0	0.000	202	-0.001	0.000	252	-0.011	-0.003
103	-0.001	0.000	153	0	0.000	203	-0.001	0.000	253	-0.007	-0.002
104	0	0.000	154	0	0.000	204	-0.001	0.000	254	-0.003	-0.001
105	0	0.000	155	0	0.000	205	-0.003	-0.001	255	-0.002	0.000
106	0	0.000	156	-0.001	0.000	206	-0.001	0.000	256	-0.001	0.000
107	0	0.000	157	-0.001	0.000	207	-0.001	0.000	257	0	0.000
108	0	0.000	158	-0.001	0.000	208	-0.001	0.000	258	0	0.000
109	-0.001	0.000	159	-0.002	0.000	209	-0.001	0.000	259	0	0.000
110	-0.001	0.000	160	-0.004	-0.001	210	0	0.000	260	0	0.000
111	-0.002	0.000	161	-0.005	-0.001	211	-0.001	0.000	261	0	0.000
112	-0.001	0.000	162	-0.008	-0.002	212	-0.002	0.000	262	0	0.000
113	-0.007	-0.002	163	-0.029	-0.007	213	-0.003	-0.001	263	0	0.000
114	-0.007	-0.002	164	-0.019	-0.005	214	-0.003	-0.001	264	0	0.000
115	-0.012	-0.003	165	-0.026	-0.006	215	-0.001	0.000	265	0	0.000
116	-0.025	-0.006	166	-0.005	-0.001	216	-0.002	0.000	266	0	0.000
117	-0.033	-0.008	167	-0.015	-0.004	217	-0.001	0.000	267	-0.001	0.000
118	-0.235	-0.056	168	-0.027	-0.006	218	-0.001	0.000	268	-0.001	0.000
119	-1.37	-0.326	169	-0.005	-0.001	219	0	0.000	269	-0.002	0.000
120	-4.582	-1.091	170	-0.003	-0.001	220	-0.001	0.000	270	-0.01	-0.002
121	-3.302	-0.786	171	-0.011	-0.003	221	0	0.000	271	-0.029	-0.007
122	-0.862	-0.205	172	-0.005	-0.001	222	0	0.000	272	-0.044	-0.010
123	-0.184	-0.044	173	-0.012	-0.003	223	0	0.000	273	-1.625	-0.387
124	-0.055	-0.013	174	-0.022	-0.005	224	0	0.000	274	-0.673	-0.160
125	-0.073	-0.017	175	-0.035	-0.008	225	0	0.000	275	-2.678	-0.638
126	-0.02	-0.005	176	-0.074	-0.018	226	0	0.000	276	-4.022	-0.958
127	-0.014	-0.003	177	-0.039	-0.009	227	0	0.000	277	-4.109	-0.978
128	-0.007	-0.002	178	-0.118	-0.028	228	0	0.000	278	-1.053	-0.251
129	-0.006	-0.001	179	-0.084	-0.020	229	-0.001	0.000	279	-0.52	-0.124
130	-0.027	-0.006	180	-0.014	-0.003	230	-0.001	0.000	280	-7.545	-1.796
131	-0.008	-0.002	181	-0.015	-0.004	231	-0.002	0.000	281	-1.83	-0.436
132	-0.065	-0.015	182	-0.015	-0.004	232	-0.002	0.000	282	-0.15	-0.036
133	-0.035	-0.008	183	-0.006	-0.001	233	-0.005	-0.001	283	-0.71	-0.169
134	-0.187	-0.045	184	-0.009	-0.002	234	-0.009	-0.002	284	-0.766	-0.182
135	-0.127	-0.030	185	-0.003	-0.001	235	-0.014	-0.003	285	-0.221	-0.053
136	-0.961	-0.229	186	-0.003	-0.001	236	-0.044	-0.010	286	-0.045	-0.011
137	-0.382	-0.091	187	-0.001	0.000	237	-0.04	-0.010	287	-0.075	-0.018
138	-0.038	-0.009	188	-0.002	0.000	238	-0.101	-0.024	288	-0.175	-0.042
139	-0.143	-0.034	189	-0.002	0.000	239	-1.68	-0.400	289	-0.033	-0.008
140	-0.016	-0.004	190	-0.003	-0.001	240	-0.499	-0.119	290	-0.444	-0.106
141	-0.014	-0.003	191	-0.005	-0.001	241	-1.671	-0.398			

Further, we aimed to find out whether electrostatic interaction energy captures the allosteric coupling in p53DBD complexes or not. The results demonstrated differential electrostatic contributions of the residues that interact strongly and favorably with the DNA (**Figure 3**). For instance, electrostatic contribution is greater than -100 kcal/mol (**Figure 3B** and **3C**) for DNA-interacting residues K120, R248, R273, and R280, whereas, iASPP binding residue H115 is stabilized by van der Waals energy contribution in p53DBD-iASPP complex (**Figure 3B** and **3C**).

More strikingly, some DNA non-interacting distal residues in p53DBD-DNA complex, e.g. R213, E258, R110 and E171, exhibit large contributions, suggesting allosteric modulation in terms of nonbonded energy. Furthermore, some residues of p53DBD undergo drastic perturbation in nonbonded energy while switching from DNA to iASPP-bound states. For example, the above mentioned DNA-binding residues show decrement in electrostatic contributions in iASPP complex compared to that of the DNA complex. On the other hand, residues K101, R110, D148, and D228 (distal from binding site) exhibit more electrostatic contributions toward iASPP than DNA. These results indicate that the above mentioned distal residues display favorable interactions in either of the complexes, alteration of which is allosterically modulated.

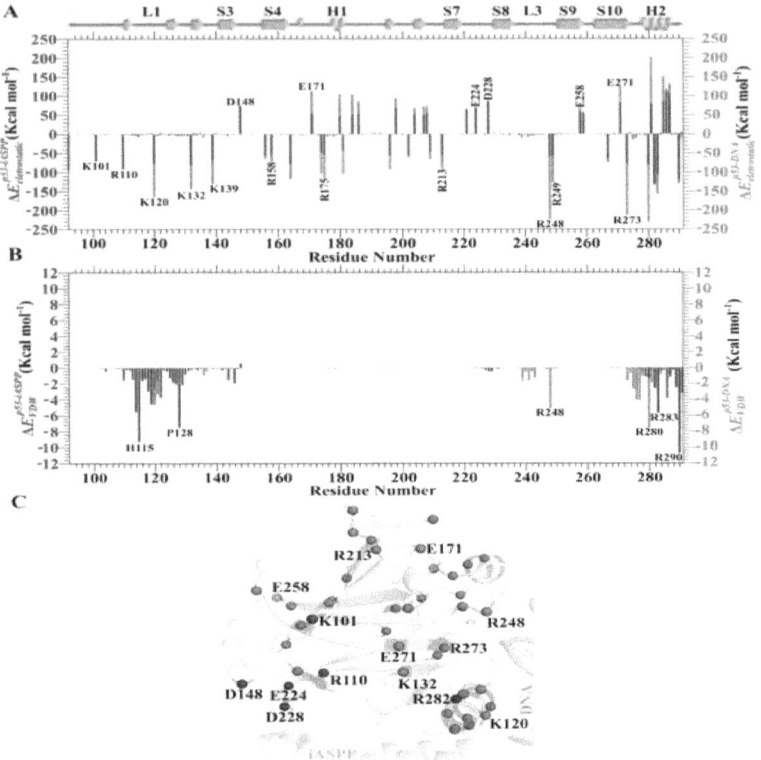

Figure 3. Residue wise contribution of nonbonded energy to DNA (red) and iASPP (blue) represented in (**A**) electrostatic contribution, (**B**) van der Waals'. Same residues of p53DBD for electrostatic contributions are used needless to say common framework for both DNA and iASPP. Most of the cases residue-wise electrostatic contribution to DNA is much higher (extended red bars) including both DNA binding and allosteric residues. Van der Waals' contributions are very less compared to electrostatic ones. (**C**) Electrostatic energy contributions for both the complexes are mapped onto representative merge crystal structure. Red spheres indicate contribution energy due to DNA binding and blue ones represent high electrostatic contributions arise upon iASPP binding. Some allosteric and binding contributions are labeled

We then considered solvent interaction energy in terms of interactions of p53DBD residues with water (cutoff distance within 2 nm) in both the complexes which shows opposite distribution patterns in the two complexes, where overall distribution is positive for DNA interaction and negative for the repressor. This is due to the dielectric effect of water which exhibits in reverse directions to the charge contributions of the residues in the form of electrostatic energy. DNA-bound complex, being more charged, shows pronounced effects compared to iASPP, where a significant amount of solvent-exposed area is shielded by the repressor. Interestingly, noticeable amount of compensation of protein-DNA electrostatic contribution energy by solvent interaction energy has been found, mainly to the main DNA-binding residues, for example, K120, R248 R273 and R280, pointing towards the incorporation of solvent molecules into the protein-DNA contact interface throughout the dynamic process of simulation. Conclusively, binding partner-dependent alterations in electrostatic contribution of p53DBD is entirely its inherent property and not due to solvation.

Electrostatic energy reveals the evolutionarily conserved allosteric communication in the complexes:

Heretofore, we have discussed the p53DBD residues that experience overall energy modulation in two different factor-bound states, using a common energy framework. Now, we closely looked into the pair-wise electrostatic interactions (ΔE_{i-j} between two intra-residues i and j of p53DBD) contributing towards these differences to generate a connectivity networkfor both the complexes (**Figure 4A-F** for p53DBD-DNA and in **Figure 4G-L** for p53DBD-iASPP complex for those residues with $|\Delta E_{i-j}| > 6$ kcal/mol, **Table 5** and **6**).[105]

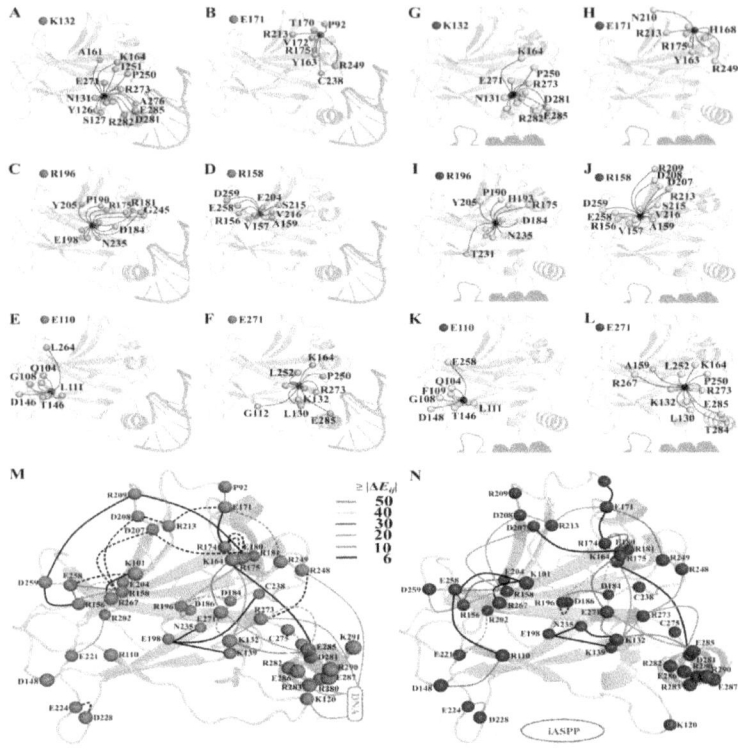

Figure 4. Allosteric crosstalk propagation in p53DBD, mediated by energy-HUBs in (**A-F**) for p53DBD-DNA and (**G-L**) for p53DBD-iASPP complex with pair-wise electrostatic interaction energy $\Delta E_{i\text{-}j}$ >6 kcal/mol. Dynamic nature of energy-HUBs can be differentiated from the distinguish extensions (by black lines) to respective differentiating residues like D207, G112, N210 etc between two complexes. Connectivity networks shown in (**M**) for DNA bound and (**N**) for iASPP bound p53DBD indicate the electrostatic energy flow between active site to allosteric region. It can be distinguished clearly the electrostatic perturbations arise due to different binding partners from the cutoff (for pair-wise electrostatic energy in kcal/mol) based color scheme. Residues for DNA and iASPP bound p53DBD are shown in red and blue spheres respectively. Dashed line indicates the lower values of the interaction energy where pair-wise energy difference between the two complexes is more than 6 kcal/mol. Significant changes among pairs E171-R249, E171-R213, R110-D148 etc. are clearly noticeable. DNA contacts are indicated by red lines. Note that, energy perturbations at allosteric sites are also prominent from different colors.

We further have defined 'energy-Hubs'. Considering residues which are electrostatically connected to large numbers of residues and participate in electrostatic energy transformation from one part to other part throughout the p53DBD energy-Hubs were defined. Considering the electrostatic betweenness-centrality approach, the same energy-Hubs were defined for p53DBD in two complexes for better comparison, namely K132, E171, R196, R158, E110 and E271 (**Figure 4A-L**). Note that, defined Hubs are evolutionarily conserved as they are conserved through various species along with p63 and p73 which indicates their real functionality.[106] Inter-energy Hubs communication is achieved in both the complexes through constituent partner residues in terms of electrostatic energy, for instance, in case of (i) p53DBD-DNA complex: hubs K132 & E171 through P250-R249 ($\Delta E_{249-250}$ = -13.5 kcal/mol); E171 & R196 through R175-R174 ($\Delta E_{174-175}$= -19 kcal/mol); R196 & R158 through E204-Y205 ($\Delta E_{204-205}$ = -19.6 kcal/mol), similarly, for (ii) p53DBD-iASPP complex: Hubs K132 & E171 through P250-R249 ($\Delta E_{249-250}$ = -13.8 kcal/mol); E171 & R196 through R175-R174 ($\Delta E_{174-175}$= -18.9 kcal/mol); R196 & R158 through E204-Y205 ($\Delta E_{204-205}$ = -21.3 kcal/mol) (**Table 5** and **6**). It is clear that for both DNA and repressor the energy Hubs are connected by the same partners in some cases with virtually same pair-wise electrostatic contributions. Nevertheless, hubs are not static in nature and distinctly different in some cases where new interacting partner residues appear exclusively in either of the complexes. For example, residues E171-C238, E110-L264, E271-G112 and K132-A161 in p53-DBD-DNA complex, and residues E171-N210, R158 with D207, D208 and R209, R196-T231, E110-E258 and E271 with A159 and R267 in p53DBD-iASPP complex. It may be noted here, most of the pair-wise interaction energies of p53DBD are higher in iASPP-bound state compared to the DNA-bound one, whereas, its energy contribution towards respective ligands is across from pair-wise interaction energy

Table 5. Residue pair-wise Electrostatic energy of p53DBD in iASPP bound state in kcal/mol

i	j	ΔE_{i-j}	i	j	ΔE_{i-j}	i	j	ΔE_{i-j}	i	j	ΔE_{i-j}
R110	L111	-33.6	R158	R156	17.3	R196	R175	10.7	E258	T155	-8.9
	F109	-9.9		V157	-11.1		H178	-6.8		R156	-37.6
	Q104	-5.2		A159	-34.5		R181	9.8		R158	-69
	G108	-10.9		E204	-9.9		D184	-57.1		E204	3.9
	W146	-9.7		S215	-5.6		D186	-14.3		T256	-3.31
	D148	-45.7		V216	-7.4		P190	-6.8		L257	-30.1
	L264	-4.3		T256	-7.7		H193	-4.7		D259	-15.5
				E258	-69		I195	-12.2		L264	-3.9
i	j	ΔE_{i-j}		D259	-3.64		V197	-31.3		L265	-3.8
R111	R110	-33.6					E198	-4		R267	-5.3
	G112	-23.4	i	j	ΔE_{i-j}		Y205	-4.7			
	T125	-3.6	E171	P92	-10.8		Y234	-4.3	i	j	ΔE_{i-j}
	Q144	-4.6		Y163	-6.2		N235	-9.7	E271	G112	4.6
	P219	-9.1		T170	-26.07		G245	8.2		L130	4
	N268	-3.04		V172	-15.4					K132	-59.1
				R174	-7.8	i	j	ΔE_{i-j}		K164	-62
i	j	ΔE_{i-j}		R213	-5.7	Y234	T140	-4.7		P250	-5.9
K132	N131	-10.6		C238	-4.1		C141	-9.1		L252	-3.1
	L130	-3.3		R249	-53.6		T155	-5.6		F270	-32.1
	Y126	-3.6					R196	-4.2		V272	-16.9
	S127	-8.3	i	j	ΔE_{i-j}		I232	-4.4		R273	-3.9
	F134	-5.9	R175	I162	-3.6		H233	-25.6		E285	20.2
	A161	4.9		R174	-19		N235	-24.5			
	K164	15.3		C176	-39.4		M246	6.5	i	j	ΔE_{i-j}
	P250	4.1		H179	-22.8				D281	K132	-6
	I251	-3.5		E180	-7.7	i	j	ΔE_{i-j}		F134	-4.9
	E271	-59.1		R181	12.5	R249	Q100	5.9		R273	-47.7
	R273	16.6		C182	-4.2		Y163	-3.8		C275	-9.39
	A276	6.2		D184	-20		K164	-3		A276	-3.6
	D281	-6		P191	-7.9		H168	-10.3		C277	-3.1
	R282	-3.1		Q192	-4.7		E171	-53.6		R280	-76.9
	E285	-68.9		H193	-5.1		V172	-3.4		R282	-9.7
				R196	10.7		G245	-4.3		R283	-5.8
i	j	ΔE_{i-j}		V216	-5.7		M246	-11.8		T284	-8.5
F270	P98	3.9		M237	8.01		N247	-4.6		E285	7.8
	N131	-5.35		G244	-6.5		R248	-15.7		R290	-4.7
	L252	-4.9		V272	3.5		P250	-13.4			
	T253	-9.7		C275	7.2						
	S269	-22.1									
	E271	-32.1									

Table 6. Residue pair-wise Electrostatic energy of p53DBD in DNA bound state in kcal/mol

i	j	$\Delta E_{i\text{-}j}$	i	j	$\Delta E_{i\text{-}j}$	i	j	$\Delta E_{i\text{-}j}$	i	j	$\Delta E_{i\text{-}j}$
R110	Q104	-16.2	L111	R110	-30.8	R196	R175	25	E258	R209	-21.8
	G108	-6.4		G112	-23.6		D184	-64.1		R158	-69
	F109	-11.2		F113	-3.2		D186	-3.1		R156	-39.8
	L111	-30.8		Q144	-4.4		P190	-6.4			
	T146	-3.4		V217	7.5		H193	-6.3	i	j	$\Delta E_{i\text{-}j}$
	D148	-67					I195	-11.9	E271	L130	4.5
	E258	8.7	i	j	$\Delta E_{i\text{-}j}$		V197	-31.7		K132	52.1
			E171	Y163	-6.9		G198	-3.5		A159	5.2
i	j	$\Delta E_{i\text{-}j}$		H168	5.3		Y205	-4.8		K164	60.6
K132	Y126	-3.4		T170	-27		T231	-6.5		P250	-4.9
	S127	-8.5		V172	-15.1		T234	-4.1		L252	-3.4
	L130	-3.7		R174	-9.3		N235	-11.2		R267	-3.07
	N131	-10.5		N210	-3.2					F270	-32.2
	M133	-35.5		R213	-19.9	i	j	$\Delta E_{i\text{-}j}$		V272	-16.8
	F134	-5.5		G245	3.7	R175	D184	-43.4		R273	-3.6
	Q136	-7.7		R249	-61.9		H179	-10		T284	-3.3
	K164	14.4								E285	16.8
	P250	4.19	i	j	$\Delta E_{i\text{-}j}$	i	j	$\Delta E_{i\text{-}j}$			
	I251	-3.6	Y234	T140	-4.7	R249	Y163	-3.5	i	j	$\Delta E_{i\text{-}j}$
	E271	-52.1		C141	-9.4		Q165	-3.7	E285	K132	-69.2
	R273	18.6		P190	5.2		H168	-14.1		F134	-3.54
	D281	-5.5		R196	-4.1		E171	-61.9		K164	-6.5
	R282	-3.4		V197	-3.1		V172	-3.7		R273	-25.3
	E285	-69.2		I232	-4.9		R174	5.1		E271	16.8
				H233	-25.7		G245	-8.2		D281	7.4
i	j	$\Delta E_{i\text{-}j}$		N235	-24.6		M246	-13.8		T284	-24.9
E286	S127	-20		L252	-4.4		N247	-7.9		E286	-23.8
	A129	-5.75					R248	-15		N288	-9.7
	L130	-4.9	i	j	$\Delta E_{i\text{-}j}$		P250	-13.8			
	R282	-68.6	R158	R156	16.7						
	R284	-7		V157	-10.7						
	R285	-23.8		A159	-34.9						
	E287	-22.7		E204	-6.4						
	L289	-7.3		D208	-18.6						
	R290	-5.81		D207	-14						
				R209	14.8						
				R213	-3.5						
				S215	-9.1						
				V216	-7.4						
				T256	-7.4						
				E258	-69						
				D259	-3.7						

We further scrutinize the residue pair-wise electrostatic contributions to intra- and inter- energy Hubs, to generate a connectivity network focusing on intra-p53DBD perturbations. Interestingly, p53DBD undergoes drastic energy perturbations in allosteric regions too (some of which are more favorable or unfavorable in either of the complexes), for both the complexes ($|\Delta E_{i\text{-}j}| > 8$

Kcal/mol). We have set electrostatic energy cut-off to differentiate the extent of perturbations (displayed in different color codes, **Figure 4M** and **4N**). In particular, residue pairs R196-D186 and R175-H179 are more favorable in DNA-bound state; whereas, R110-D148, E171-R213, R175-D184 and E171-R249 are more favorable in iASPP-bound complex. Notably, the above mentioned residues are connected to each other either by salt-bridges or hydrogen bonding as confirmed by respective crystal structures.

In both the complexes, a distant residue R213 is connected to DNA-binding residue R248 through the evolutionarily conserved path: R248=>R249=>E171=>R213 (**Figure 5A** and **5B**).

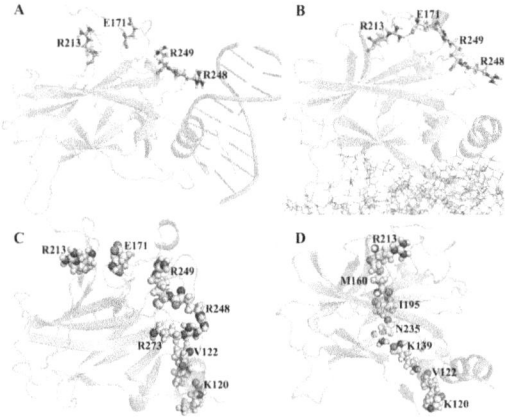

Figure 5. Representative snapshots showing comparison of communication path mapped on (A) DNA bound and (B) iASPP bound p53DBD structure that transfers the signal from DNA binding active site to allosteric site in form of electrostatic energy. Residues are shown in stick. Broken hydrogen bonds are shown to visualize the transcriptionally active p53DBD in DNA bound state only. Loop L1 conformation mediated dynamic electrostatic path of (C) DNA bound and (D) iASPP bound p53 connecting residue K120 to R213. To show the path difference constituent residues are labeled. All residues are shown in sphere.

Note that, R213 is the frequently mutated amino acid site in endocrine cancers.[107] Interestingly, when compared to respective crystal structures, it is clear that the R213-E171 H-bond retains in iASPP-bound p53DBD through which allosteric cross-talk propagates. On the contrary, R213-E171 H-bond breaks in DNA bound state. In this context, it may be noted here that in the p53 complex with tumor suppressor p53-binding protein 1 (53BP1), the H-bond between E171-R249 is disrupted making the NH1 and NH2 groups of R249 free to interact with 53BP1.[108]

The above-discussed path connects DNA-binding surface to distal (allosteric) region of p53DBD. However, the same path does not connect the iASPP binding interface to the allosteric site. Thus, we have chosen a common interface to both DNA and repressor, residue K120 of the L1 loop region and distal residue R213. Selection of these residues for determining the dynamic path is reasonable since the key role played by the repressor iASPP is to shift L1 loop away from helix H2, as revealed by the crystal structures. As a consequence of this shift, we revealed that communication follows different paths in the two complexes (**Figure 5C** and **5D**). Note that, in DNA complex this path is actually the extension of previously mentioned evolutionarily conserved path and though both paths from common interface are different but both consist of evolutionarily conserved residues.[106]

Analysis of the path in the DNA-bound complex allowed us to correlate dynamicity and electrostatic energy. In DCCM calculation for DNA, reported in earlier section, moderate correlation among DNA-binding residues. In agreement with that result, the path between K120-R213 successfully set R273, R248 as milestones. The cross-correlation disappears in iASPP complex, as the path through DNA-bonding residues switches to other constituent residues following repressor binding.

Pair-wise side-chain distance population shift modulates energy perturbations and manipulates side-chain conformational entropy:

So far we have shown significant differential electrostatic perturbation of the residues in two different complexes of p53DBD. To understand the underlying reason behind this observation we have calculated pairwise distance distribution of those residues throughout the trajectory (**Figure 6F-N**). It is clear that most of the pairs show population peaks around 0.2 nm (hydrogen atoms are not indexed here for calculation), clearly indicating H-bond or salt bridge-mediated connections within the pairs. The crystal structure of iASPP-bound p53 shows H-bond between E171-R213 residues. The single population peak without any shoulder (**Figure 6G**) for iASPP-bound p53 complex reestablished the existence of this state. Significantly, population peak of this pair (around 0.2 nm) almost disappeared in the DNA-bound complex (**Figure 6G**), in agreement with the crystal structure which shows breakage of H-bond in E171-R213 pair upon DNA-binding (**Figure 6C and D**).

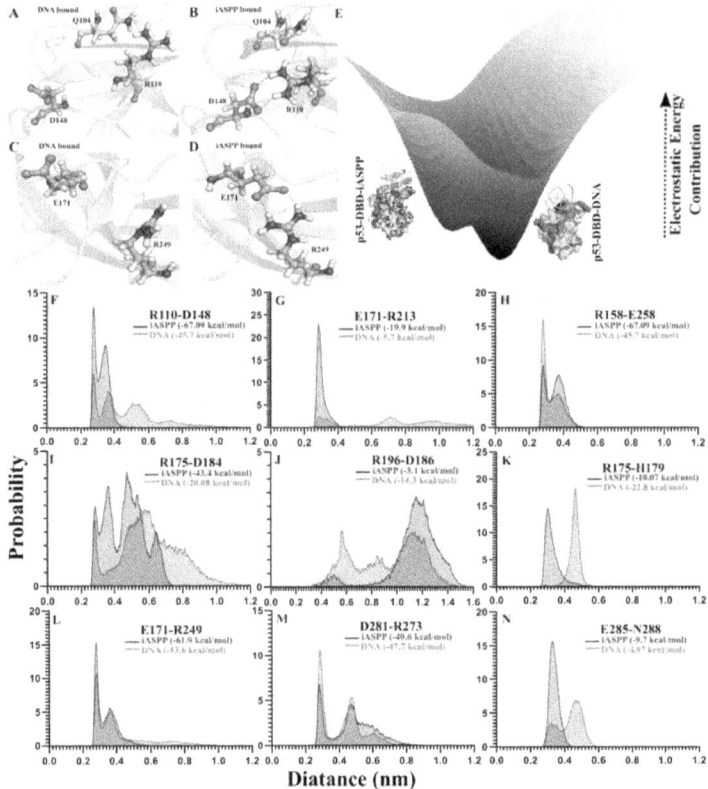

Figure 6. Snapshots representing hydrogen bond breakage, precisely the enhancement of entropy in side chains where (**A&C**) and (**B&D**) actually represent allosteric rearrangement of sidechains in DNA and iASPP bound p53DBD. (**C**) Schematic of electrostatic contribution energy landscape for both the complexes. (**F-N**) Comparison of probability distribution of pairwise distance throughout the trajectory of p53DBD residues bound to both DNA (red) and iASPP (blue). Corresponding pairwise interaction energy has been given with corresponding color codes.

Peaks around 0.2 nm (Hydrogen atoms are not included in calculation) represent existence of H-bonds or salt bridges.

In the DCCM profile we have found correlated motions appear due to DNA binding which is missing in case of repressor-bound state. In the case of R175-H179 pair, DNA binding-mediated rearrangement occurs with shift in population (**Figure 6K**), which is missing in the iASPP-bound complex validating our cross-correlation analysis. The results also reinforce the previous reports showing removal of Zinc ion abolishes site-specific DNA-binding activity by fluorescence anisotropy,[109,110] whereas, R175H substitution causes enhancement of iASPP binding.

Conclusively, the energy perturbation is strongly correlated to population shift with respect to distance and in most of the cases it is determined by H-bonding. This can also be correlated to either enhancement of conformational entropy upon DNA-binding, where pairwise energy decreases by relaxing H-bonds (side-chain contribution is more dominating) or decrement of the same due to iASPP binding, where strengthening of H-bonding increases the pairwise energy.

We have shown that binding partner-dependent modulation of electrostatic energy plays a crucial role to stabilize p53DBD in the energy landscape. The overall residue-wise electrostatic contribution towards DNA is much more negative (than that of iASPP) compared to intra-residue pairwise interaction energy of p53DBD. Notably, in DNA-bound state, pairwise interaction energy decreases due to distance population shift in the form of breakage of H-bond or salt bridge indicating enhanced plasticity (randomness in the form of conformational entropy) of side-chains. Despite the fact that the same electrostatic energy framework is shared by p53DBD in molecular recognition of either DNA or repressor, the ligand-dependent electrostatic energy contribution varies, reflecting on thermodynamic enthalpy changes towards the free energy of binding. It is evident that evolutionarily conserved energy-hubs are utilized to relay information throughout p53DBD using substrate-dependent dynamicity of p53DBD. For the DNA-binding domain (p53DBD) of tumor suppressor p53 (being the 'guardian of genome') it is necessary to interact with other cofactors in its DNA-bound state during transcription and decrease in pairwise interactions is required in this case (H-bond breakage). On the other hand, formation or strengthening of H-bonds makes p53DBD which is also well justified with enhanced pair-wise interaction energies of the same, as inferred from our calculations, and iASPP plays the role successfully (Movie S1). In other words, factor-dependent (e.g. DNA, repressors etc.) energy perturbation is necessary for p53DBD to capture it in a specific conformational state corresponding to a 'valley' in the energy landscape.

Taken together, in this study we have dissected p53DBD into residue level to analyze electrostatic contributions toward ligands and pair-wise interaction energies along with van der Waals' and solvation energy, which have not been highlighted earlier for p53. Furthermore, we have reported the biologically relevant evolutionarily conserved communication connecting the allosteric site to the active site and the inherent energy flow-network which would be highly significant in the field of target-specific orthosteric as well as allosteric drug designing.The tumor suppressor protein p53 is one of the most essential proteins considered as a key target for designing cancer therapeutics. The present study, by providing residue wise energy information, would have a significant impact on the drug designing field where cell context-dependent p53 alteration is critical for the life-or-death balance.

Chapter - IV

Structural and functional characterization of both full-length wild type and P152L p53

Background and Objective

In this section, a structural comparison between the wild-type (WT) full length (FL) p53 and a Gain-of-Function (GOF) mutant P152L was performed. P152L, a GOF mutant which was not characterized previously either in structural or functional aspects. Due to the P152L mutation, the DBD of the mutant p53 binds more strongly to RE but the FL mutant loses its binding affinity completely.[111] In this chapter, the global conformational change of FL-P152L-p53 with respect to WT p53 was characterized by structural techniques.

Materials and Methods

Expression and Purification of FL-p53:

N-terminal His-tagged p53 gene was inserted in the pET15b vector. The transformation was done in E. coli BL21 (DE3), and the protein was expressed for 16 h at 15°C. Lysis was done in a 20 mM Tris-HCl buffer, pH 8.0, containing 150 mM NaCl and purified with 100-250 mM an imidazole gradient. Further purification was done in AKTA PURE FPLC with a 16/600 Superdex-200pg (GE Healthcare) at 4°C.

Atomic force microscopy (AFM):

Purified FL-p53 was transferred to PBS through buffer exchange and morphological changes due to mutation were visualized with Acoustic AC (AAC) Atomic Force Microscopy (AFM) using a Pico plus 5500 AFM (Agilent Technologies, USA) with a piezo-scanner having a maximum range of 9 μm. The images were processed using Pico view 1.12 software (Agilent Technologies, USA).

Transmission electron microscopy (TEM):

Buffer exchanged samples were loaded to a carbon-coated copper grid (300-mesh), followed by staining with 2% uranyl acetate. Imaging was done using a FEI Tecnai-12 BioTwin Transmission Electron Microscope at NICED, Kolkata.

Cryogenic electron microscopy (Cryo-EM):

For cryo-EM, 4 µL of P152L p53 was applied on glow-discharged Quantifoil holey carbon transmission electron microscopy (TEM) grids (R2/2, Quantifoil, Micro Tools GmbH), followed by blotting and vitrification with a Vitrobot (FEI Inc.) and then frozen in liquid ethane. Initial Cryo-EM data were acquired at IICB in Tecnai Polara microscope (FEI, USA) equipped with a FEG (Field Emission Gun) operating at 300 kV. Images were collected with 4K X 4K 'Eagle' charge-coupled device (CCD) camera (FEI, USA) at ~79000X magnification, resulting in a pixel size 1.89 Å at the specimen level with defocus values ranging from 1.5 to 4.5µm, and processed with EMAN2 package with a preliminary of 16Å.

Dynamic light scattering (DLS):

Dynamic light scattering measurements were recorded at room temperature for both FL-WT and FL-P152L p53 in 20 mM Tris-HCl buffer, pH 8.0 containing 150 mM NaCl and 100 µM ZnCl2 at a concentration of 1 µM with a Zetasizer Nano ZS (Malvern Instruments, U.K.) equipped with 4 mW He–Ne laser source (λ=632.8 nm) and a detector positioned at a scattering angle of 173°. Scattering data were collected as an average of three measurements with 20 scans for each measurement.

Denaturation experiment:

Purified proteins were dialyzed against 20 mM Tris-HCl buffer, pH 8.0 containing 150 mM NaCl and 100 µM ZnCl2 and concentrated with Amicon® Ultra-15 100 kDa Centrifugal Filter Units up to 2 µM for each FL-WT and FL-P152L p53.

For denaturation experiments, protein samples were incubated overnight (approximately 18 h) at 25°C at increasing concentrations of GuHCl (0.25 M-6 M) (G3272, Sigma-Aldrich). Intrinsic tryptophan fluorescence intensity was measured at 25°C using a Hitachi F-7000 FL Spectrophotometer (ex: 295 nm; em: 310- 450 nm; ex/em slit widths 5 nm; at 2400 nm/min). The fluorescence intensities of corresponding solutions without protein samples were subtracted as background from each reading. The measurements were performed in triplicates, with each dataset consisting of an average of four individual scans.

Isothermal Titration Calorimetry (ITC):

WT p53 at 100 nM concentration was titrated against 2 µM of a duplex oligodeoxynucleotide containing the GADD45 response element at 25°C at the interval of 240 sec in each injection with MicroCal VP-ITC unit (MicroCal, Inc.; Northampton, MA, USA).

Results and Discussion:

ITC data (**Figure 1A**) and negatively stained image (**Figure 1B**) of WT FL p53 clearly indicates the formation of tetramer as the functionally active species for DNA binding.

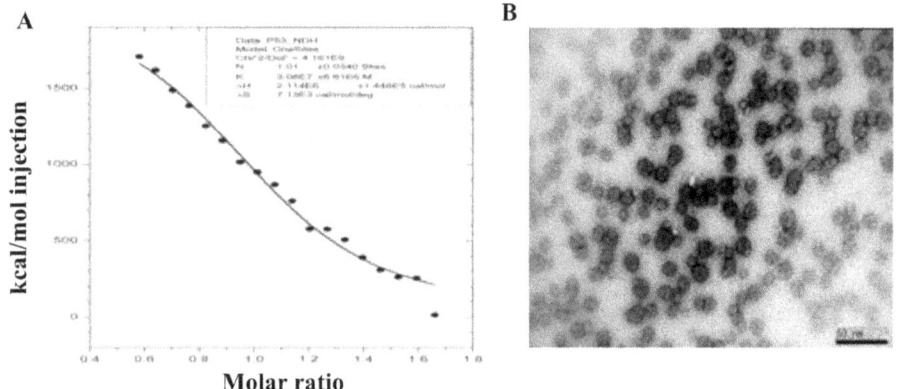

Figure 1: Functional characterisation of WT p53 with ITC. (A) Tetrameric p53 unit binds to GADD45 DNA RE. **(B) Structural characterization of WT p53 with TEM.** Negatively stained tetrameric p53.

For structural insights into both WT and P152L p53, initial screening was done with AFM indicating the structural differences with respect to both tetramerizationand fibril formation

(**Figure 2**). WTFL p53 showed much more homogeneity compared to the P152L p53. Similarly, WT p53 formed fibril but at the same condition P152L showed no fibrillation.

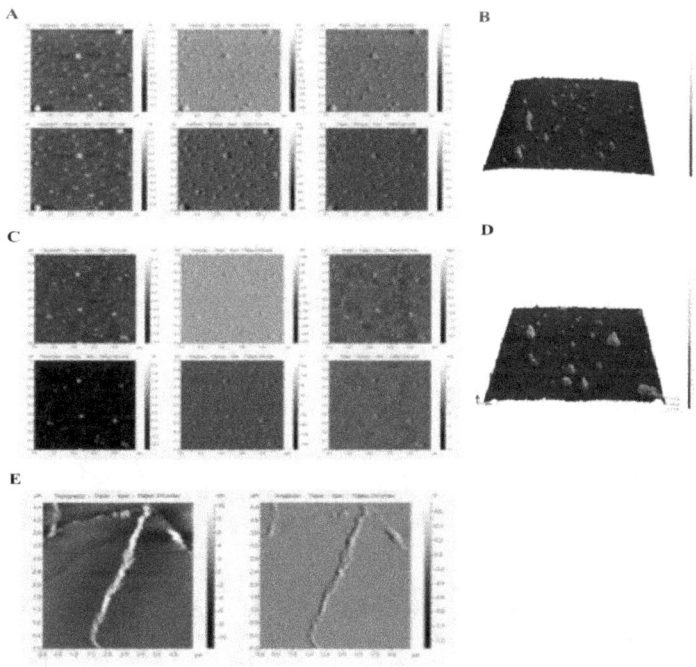

Figure 2: Structural characterization with AFM: (A) WT-FL p53 (C) P152L-FL p53 (D) Fibril formation by P152L which was not found in WT FL p53. 3D representations are shown in (B) for WT-FL p53 and (D) for P152L-FL p53.

Cryo-EM is the most suitable tool to demonstrate intrinsically flexible macromolecules. However, so far no high-resolution cryo-EM structure of p53 is available. Evidently, it is not easy to generate cryo-EM structure of the protein tetramer, possibly due to structural heterogeneity. For cryo-EM study of P152L p53, I have employed single particle 3D reconstruction technique. To this end, I have collected 110 number of cryo-EM micrographs. A 3D density map was generated from 11580 number of particles. The 2D averages show tetramer features (**Figure 3C**). The resolution of the 3D map was limited. However, when compared with the existing WT p53 map (~13.7Å resolution),[112] it shows the basis for its functional plasticity as a tetramer. Further structural comparison between WT and P152L was monitored with cryo-EM single particle 3D reconstruction, which shows some extra density in P152L compared with WT p53 though it was not possible to achieve higher resolution (**Figure 3B and D**). Hence, specific conclusion can not be obtained from this but this structure could be a good stating point for future higher resolution structure determination from cryo-EM of P152L-FL p53.

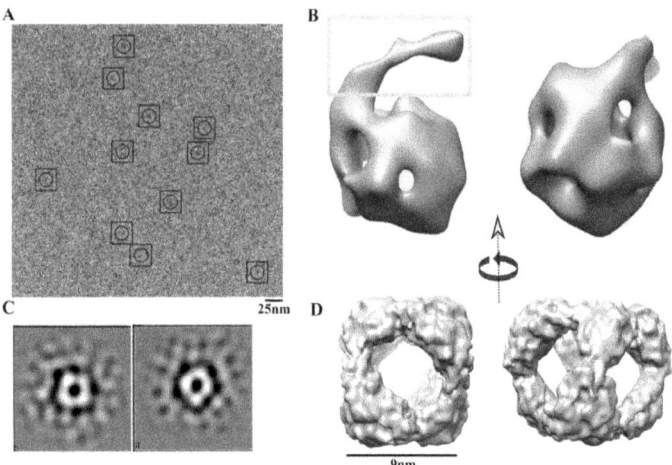

Figure 3: Structural characterization of P152L p53 with Cryo-EM. (A) Micrograph showing selected particles in blue box.(B) 3D model (reconstruction was done by picking small number of particles). Differential density was marked within green box. (C) 2D classification of P152L p53 and (D) Published structure of WT p53 (EMD: 1141).

Further validation in overall structure and stability was done with DSC (**Figure 4**) and denaturation experiment (**Figure 5**) are clearly indicating that in solution there are quaternary structural differences on the basis of hydrodynamic radius and intra-domain connectivity. the DLS profile of the wild-type and P152Lp53. The measured hydrodynamic radii are 35.5 Å and 40.9 Å, respectively for the wild-type and P152Lp53.

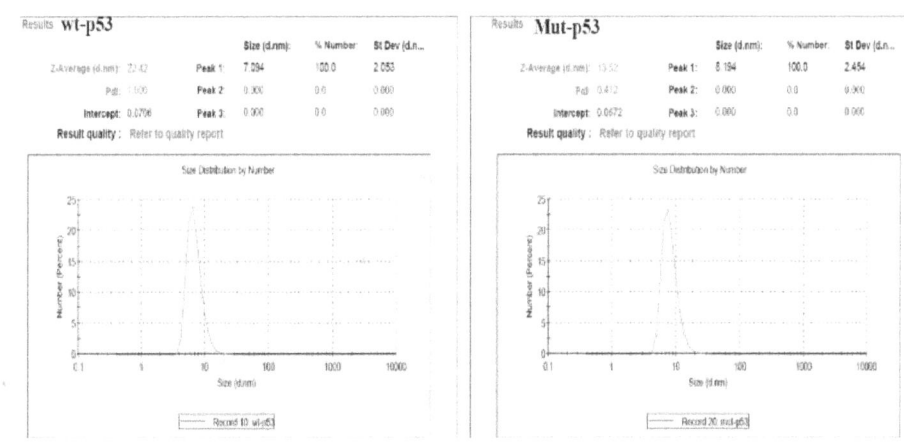

Figure 4: Measurement of Hydrodynamic radii with DLS. The wild-type p53 has a hydrodynamic radius of 35.5 Å and the mutant p53 has a radius of 40.9 Å.

The measured radiisuggest that neither of the proteins is aggregated to any significant extent and the P152Lp53 protein is modestly enlarged. This is consistent with the idea that the subunits are arranged in a different mode in the mutant protein. GuHCl (Guanidine Hydrochloride) denaturation of the wild-type and mutant tetramers was performed to measure the stability of the proteins. **Figure5** shows the GuHCl-induced equilibrium denaturation profile of the wild-type and P152Lp53 asmeasured by increased solvent exposure of tryptophan residues (F340/F350) as a function ofGuHCl. The fitted curve is a two-state equation as described earlier.[113]

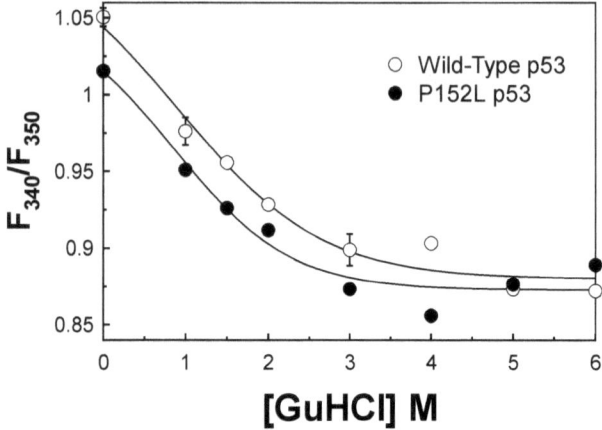

Figure 5: Equilibrium GuHCl denaturation of Wild-Type and P152L p53. The data is fitted in a two-state equation. Each data point is an average of three independent biological replicates.

The fluorescence emission spectra of the mutant are modestly red-shifted compared to that of the wild-type (reflected in the lower F340/F350 value of the mutant). The mid-points of the transition of the wild-type and the mutant protein are around 1.1 M GuHCl, indicating the stability is not impacted by the mutation in a major way. Taken together, both WT and P152L p53 behaves differently and the high resolution descriptions of WT and mutant p53 can shed light on the differences in functional behavior of the two.

References

1. Parkin, D. M., Bray, F., Ferlay, J. & Pisani, P. Global cancer statistics, 2002. *CA Cancer J. Clin.* **55**, 74–108 (2005).

2. Feinberg, A. P. & Tycko, B. The history of cancer epigenetics. *Nat. Rev. Cancer* **4**, 143–153 (2004).

3. Hanahan, D. & Weinberg, R. A. The Hallmarks of Cancer. *Cell* vol. 100 57–70 (2000).

4. Krepulat, F. *et al.* Epigenetic mechanisms affect mutant p53 transgene expression in WAP-mutp53 transgenic mice. *Oncogene* **24**, 4645–4659 (2005).

5. Stracquadanio, G. *et al.* The importance of p53 pathway genetics in inherited and somatic cancer genomes. *Nat. Rev. Cancer* **16**, 251–265 (2016).

6. Lane, D. P. & Crawford, L. V. T antigen is bound to a host protein in SV40-transformed cells. *Nature* **278**, 261–263 (1979).

7. DeLeo, A. B. *et al.* Detection of a transformation-related antigen in chemically induced sarcomas and other transformed cells of the mouse. *Proc. Natl. Acad. Sci. U. S. A.* **76**, 2420–2424 (1979).

8. Finley, R. S. Lung cancer: detection, prevention, and therapeutics. *Am. Pharm.* **NS29**, 39–46 (1989).

9. Nigro, J. M. *et al.* Mutations in the p53 gene occur in diverse human tumour types. *Nature* **342**, 705–708 (1989).

10. Bourdon, J.-C. *et al.* p53 isoforms can regulate p53 transcriptional activity. *Genes Dev.* **19**, 2122–2137 (2005).

11. Reisman, D., Greenberg, M. & Rotter, V. Human p53 oncogene contains one promoter upstream of exon 1 and a second, stronger promoter within intron 1. *Proc. Natl. Acad. Sci. U. S. A.* **85**, 5146–5150 (1988).

12. Nikolova, P. V. Mechanism of rescue of common p53 cancer mutations by second-site suppressor mutations. *The EMBO Journal* vol. 19 370–378 (2000).
13. May, P. & May, E. Twenty years of p53 research: structural and functional aspects of the p53 protein. *Oncogene* 18, 7621–7636 (1999).
14. Soussi, T., Caron de Fromentel, C. & May, P. Structural aspects of the p53 protein in relation to gene evolution. *Oncogene* 5, 945–952 (1990).
15. Brady, C. A. *et al.* Distinct p53 transcriptional programs dictate acute DNA-damage responses and tumor suppression. *Cell* 145, 571–583 (2011).
16. Sakamuro, D., Sabbatini, P., White, E. & Prendergast, G. C. The polyproline region of p53 is required to activate apoptosis but not growth arrest. *Oncogene* 15, 887–898 (1997).
17. Cho, Y., Gorina, S., Jeffrey, P. D. & Pavletich, N. P. Crystal structure of a p53 tumor suppressor-DNA complex: understanding tumorigenic mutations. *Science* 265, 346–355 (1994).
18. Shaulsky, G., Goldfinger, N., Ben-Ze'ev, A. & Rotter, V. Nuclear accumulation of p53 protein is mediated by several nuclear localization signals and plays a role in tumorigenesis. *Mol. Cell. Biol.* 10, 6565–6577 (1990).
19. Pietenpol, J. A. *et al.* Sequence-specific transcriptional activation is essential for growth suppression by p53. *Proc. Natl. Acad. Sci. U. S. A.* 91, 1998–2002 (1994).
20. Wang, Y. & Prives, C. Increased and altered DNA binding of human p53 by S and G2/M but not G1 cyclin-dependent kinases. *Nature* 376, 88–91 (1995).
21. Joerger, A. C. & Fersht, A. R. Structural biology of the tumor suppressor p53. *Annu. Rev. Biochem.* 77, 557–582 (2008).
22. el-Deiry, W. S., Kern, S. E., Pietenpol, J. A., Kinzler, K. W. & Vogelstein, B. Definition of a consensus binding site for p53. *Nat. Genet.* 1, 45–49 (1992).
23. Joruiz, S. M. & Bourdon, J.-C. p53 Isoforms: Key Regulators of the Cell Fate Decision.

Cold Spring Harb. Perspect. Med. **6**, (2016).

24. Joerger, A. C. & Bauer, M. Crystal structure of the p53 cancer mutant Y220C in complex with a monofluorinated derivative of the small molecule stabilizer Phikan083. (2016) doi:10.2210/pdb5g4m/pdb.

25. Lavin, M. F. & Gueven, N. The complexity of p53 stabilization and activation. *Cell Death Differ.* **13**, 941–950 (2006).

26. Lakin, N. D. & Jackson, S. P. Regulation of p53 in response to DNA damage. *Oncogene* **18**, 7644–7655 (1999).

27. Maddocks, O. D. K. & Vousden, K. H. Erratum to: Metabolic regulation by p53. *Journal of Molecular Medicine* vol. 89 531–531 (2011).

28. Arsic, N. *et al.* The p53 isoform Δ133p53β promotes cancer stem cell potential. *Stem Cell Reports* **4**, 531–540 (2015).

29. Liu, J., Zhang, C., Zhao, Y. & Feng, Z. MicroRNA Control of p53. *Journal of Cellular Biochemistry* vol. 118 7–14 (2017).

30. Momand, J., Zambetti, G. P., Olson, D. C., George, D. & Levine, A. J. The mdm-2 oncogene product forms a complex with the p53 protein and inhibits p53-mediated transactivation. *Cell* **69**, 1237–1245 (1992).

31. Oliner, J. D. *et al.* Oncoprotein MDM2 conceals the activation domain of tumour suppressor p53. *Nature* **362**, 857–860 (1993).

32. Gottifredi, V. & Prives, C. Molecular biology. Getting p53 out of the nucleus. *Science* vol. 292 1851–1852 (2001).

33. Juven, T., Barak, Y., Zauberman, A., George, D. L. & Oren, M. Wild type p53 can mediate sequence-specific transactivation of an internal promoter within the mdm2 gene. *Oncogene* **8**, 3411–3416 (1993).

34. Dornan, D. *et al.* Interferon regulatory factor 1 binding to p300 stimulates DNA-dependent

acetylation of p53. *Mol. Cell. Biol.* **24**, 10083–10098 (2004).

35. Canman, C. E. & Kastan, M. B. Small contribution of G1 checkpoint control manipulation to modulation of p53-mediated apoptosis. *Oncogene* **16**, 957–966 (1998).

36. Drainas, A. P. *et al.* Genome-wide Screens Implicate Loss of Cullin Ring Ligase 3 in Persistent Proliferation and Genome Instability in TP53-Deficient Cells. *Cell Rep.* **31**, 107465 (2020).

37. Baudier, J., Delphin, C., Grunwald, D., Khochbin, S. & Lawrence, J. J. Characterization of the tumor suppressor protein p53 as a protein kinase C substrate and a S100b-binding protein. *Proc. Natl. Acad. Sci. U. S. A.* **89**, 11627–11631 (1992).

38. Vousden, K. H. & Lu, X. Live or let die: the cell's response to p53. *Nat. Rev. Cancer* **2**, 594–604 (2002).

39. Di Stefano, V., Rinaldo, C., Sacchi, A., Soddu, S. & D'Orazi, G. Homeodomain-interacting protein kinase-2 activity and p53 phosphorylation are critical events for cisplatin-mediated apoptosis. *Exp. Cell Res.* **293**, 311–320 (2004).

40. Barlev, N. A. *et al.* Acetylation of p53 activates transcription through recruitment of coactivators/histone acetyltransferases. *Mol. Cell* **8**, 1243–1254 (2001).

41. O'Brate, A., Tarón, M., Gandara, D. & Rosell, R. Sharing new approaches to translational research in non-small cell lung cancer. *Oncologist* **5**, 514–519 (2000).

42. Liang, S. H. & Clarke, M. F. The nuclear import of p53 is determined by the presence of a basic domain and its relative position to the nuclear localization signal. *Oncogene* **18**, 2163–2166 (1999).

43. Stommel, J. M. *et al.* A leucine-rich nuclear export signal in the p53 tetramerization domain: regulation of subcellular localization and p53 activity by NES masking. *EMBO J.* **18**, 1660–1672 (1999).

44. Zhang, M., Li, Y., Zhang, H. & Xue, S. APOPTOSIS. vol. 6 291–297 (2001).

45. Yu, Z. K., Geyer, R. K. & Maki, C. G. MDM2-dependent ubiquitination of nuclear and cytoplasmic P53. *Oncogene* **19**, 5892–5897 (2000).

46. Soussi, T. p53 Protein, biological and clinical aspects. *Encyclopedic Reference of Cancer* 669–675 doi:10.1007/3-540-30683-8_1256.

47. Bullock, A. N. & Fersht, A. R. Rescuing the function of mutant p53. *Nature Reviews Cancer* vol. 1 68–76 (2001).

48. Soussi, T. & Béroud, C. Assessing TP53 status in human tumours to evaluate clinical outcome. *Nat. Rev. Cancer* **1**, 233–240 (2001).

49. Lowe, S. W., Schmitt, E. M., Smith, S. W., Osborne, B. A. & Jacks, T. p53 is required for radiation-induced apoptosis in mouse thymocytes. *Nature* **362**, 847–849 (1993).

50. Stad, R. *et al.* Mdmx stabilizes p53 and Mdm2 via two distinct mechanisms. *EMBO Rep.* **2**, 1029–1034 (2001).

51. Chen, L. & Chen, J. MDM2-ARF complex regulates p53 sumoylation. *Oncogene* **22**, 5348–5357 (2003).

52. Sengupta, S., Vonesch, J. L., Waltzinger, C., Zheng, H. & Wasylyk, B. Negative cross-talk between p53 and the glucocorticoid receptor and its role in neuroblastoma cells. *EMBO J.* **19**, 6051–6064 (2000).

53. Wang, G. & Fersht, A. R. Mechanism of initiation of aggregation of p53 revealed by Φ-value analysis. *Proc. Natl. Acad. Sci. U. S. A.* **112**, 2437–2442 (2015).

54. Ano Bom, A. P. D. *et al.* Mutant p53 aggregates into prion-like amyloid oligomers and fibrils: implications for cancer. *J. Biol. Chem.* **287**, 28152–28162 (2012).

55. Wu, L., Ma, C. A. & Jain, A. When Aurora B met p53: newly revealed regulatory phosphorylation in an old protein. *Cell Cycle* **10**, 171–172 (2011).

56. Popovych, N., Tzeng, S. R. & Kalodimos, C. G. Nmr structure of catabolite activator protein in the unliganded state. (2009) doi:10.2210/pdb2wc2/pdb.

57. Oren, M. & Rotter, V. Mutant p53 gain-of-function in cancer. *Cold Spring Harb. Perspect. Biol.* **2**, a001107 (2010).

58. Tzeng, S.-R. & Kalodimos, C. G. The role of slow and fast protein motions in allosteric interactions. *Biophys. Rev.* **7**, 251–255 (2015).

59. Froger, A. & Hall, J. E. Transformation of plasmid DNA into E. coli using the heat shock method. *J. Vis. Exp.* 253 (2007).

60. Delaglio, F. *et al.* NMRPipe: a multidimensional spectral processing system based on UNIX pipes. *J. Biomol. NMR* **6**, 277–293 (1995).

61. Lee, W., Westler, W. M., Bahrami, A., Eghbalnia, H. R. & Markley, J. L. PINE-SPARKY: graphical interface for evaluating automated probabilistic peak assignments in protein NMR spectroscopy. *Bioinformatics* vol. 25 2085–2087 (2009).

62. Mandel, A. M., Akke, M., Palmer, A. G. & III. Backbone Dynamics ofEscherichia coliRibonuclease HI: Correlations with Structure and Function in an Active Enzyme. *Journal of Molecular Biology* vol. 246 144–163 (1995).

63. Tjandra, N. & Bax, A. Direct measurement of distances and angles in biomolecules by NMR in a dilute liquid crystalline medium. *Science* **278**, 1111–1114 (1997).

64. Tjandra, N., Omichinski, J. G., Gronenborn, A. M., Clore, G. M. & Bax, A. Use of dipolar 1H-15N and 1H-13C couplings in the structure determination of magnetically oriented macromolecules in solution. *Nat. Struct. Biol.* **4**, 732–738 (1997).

65. Lipari, G. & Szabo, A. ChemInform Abstract: MODEL-FREE APPROACH TO THE INTERPRETATION OF NUCLEAR MAGNETIC RESONANCE RELAXATION IN MACROMOLECULES. 2. ANALYSIS OF EXPERIMENTAL RESULTS. *Chemischer Informationsdienst* vol. 13 (1982).

66. Cole, R. & Loria, J. P. FAST-Modelfree: a program for rapid automated analysis of solution NMR spin-relaxation data. *J. Biomol. NMR* **26**, 203–213 (2003).

67. Yang, D. & Kay, L. E. Contributions to Conformational Entropy Arising from Bond Vector Fluctuations Measured from NMR-Derived Order Parameters: Application to Protein Folding. *Journal of Molecular Biology* vol. 263 369–382 (1996).

68. Lindorff-Larsen, K. et al. Improved side-chain torsion potentials for the Amber ff99SB protein force field. *Proteins* **78**, 1950–1958 (2010).

69. Spoel, D. V. D. et al. GROMACS: Fast, flexible, and free. *Journal of Computational Chemistry* vol. 26 1701–1718 (2005).

70. Rostkowski, M., Olsson, M. H. M., Søndergaard, C. R. & Jensen, J. H. Graphical analysis of pH-dependent properties of proteins predicted using PROPKA. *BMC Struct. Biol.* **11**, 6 (2011).

71. Price, D. J. & Brooks, C. L., 3rd. A modified TIP3P water potential for simulation with Ewald summation. *J. Chem. Phys.* **121**, 10096–10103 (2004).

72. Ghosh, A. & Vishveshwara, S. A study of communication pathways in methionyl- tRNA synthetase by molecular dynamics simulations and structure network analysis. *Proc. Natl. Acad. Sci. U. S. A.* **104**, 15711–15716 (2007).

73. Jeong, H., Mason, S. P., Barabási, A. L. & Oltvai, Z. N. Lethality and centrality in protein networks. *Nature* **411**, 41–42 (2001).

74. Patil, A. & Nakamura, H. Disordered domains and high surface charge confer hubs with the ability to interact with multiple proteins in interaction networks. *FEBS Lett.* **580**, 2041–2045 (2006).

75. Shammas, S. L. Mechanistic roles of protein disorder within transcription. *Curr. Opin. Struct. Biol.* **42**, 155–161 (2017).

76. Farnebo, M., Bykov, V. J. N. & Wiman, K. G. The p53 tumor suppressor: a master regulator of diverse cellular processes and therapeutic target in cancer. *Biochem. Biophys. Res. Commun.* **396**, 85–89 (2010).

77. Mello, S. S. & Attardi, L. D. Deciphering p53 signaling in tumor suppression. *Curr. Opin. Cell Biol.* **51**, 65–72 (2018).

78. Aylon, Y. & Oren, M. The Paradox of p53: What, How, and Why? *Cold Spring Harb. Perspect. Med.* **6**, (2016).

79. Tuncbag, N., Kar, G., Gursoy, A., Keskin, O. & Nussinov, R. Towards inferring time dimensionality in protein-protein interaction networks by integrating structures: the p53 example. *Mol. Biosyst.* **5**, 1770–1778 (2009).

80. Sykes, S. M. *et al.* Acetylation of the p53 DNA-binding domain regulates apoptosis induction. *Mol. Cell* **24**, 841–851 (2006).

81. Lakomek, N.-A., Ying, J. & Bax, A. Measurement of ^{15}N relaxation rates in perdeuterated proteins by TROSY-based methods. *J. Biomol. NMR* **53**, 209–221 (2012).

82. Hansen, A. L., Lundström, P., Velyvis, A. & Kay, L. E. Quantifying millisecond exchange dynamics in proteins by CPMG relaxation dispersion NMR using side-chain 1H probes. *J. Am. Chem. Soc.* **134**, 3178–3189 (2012).

83. Huart, A.-S. & Hupp, T. Evolution of Conformational Disorder & Diversity of the P53 Interactome. *Biodiscovery* 5 (2013).

84. Inoue, K., Fry, E. A. & Frazier, D. P. Transcription factors that interact with p53 and Mdm2. *Int. J. Cancer* **138**, 1577–1585 (2016).

85. Chen, S. *et al.* iASPP mediates p53 selectivity through a modular mechanism fine-tuning DNA recognition. *Proc. Natl. Acad. Sci. U. S. A.* **116**, 17470–17479 (2019).

86. Robinson, R. A., Lu, X., Jones, E. Y. & Siebold, C. Biochemical and structural studies of ASPP proteins reveal differential binding to p53, p63, and p73. *Structure* **16**, 259–268 (2008).

87. Kitayner, M. *et al.* Structural basis of DNA recognition by p53 tetramers. *Mol. Cell* **22**, 741–753 (2006).

88. Kumawat, A. & Chakrabarty, S. Hidden electrostatic basis of dynamic allostery in a PDZ domain. *Proceedings of the National Academy of Sciences* vol. 114 E5825–E5834 (2017).

89. Georgescu, R. E., Alexov, E. G. & Gunner, M. R. Combining conformational flexibility and continuum electrostatics for calculating pK(a)s in proteins. *Biophys. J.* **83**, 1731–1748 (2002).

90. Olsson, M. H. M., Søndergaard, C. R., Rostkowski, M. & Jensen, J. H. PROPKA3: Consistent Treatment of Internal and Surface Residues in Empirical pKa Predictions. *J. Chem. Theory Comput.* **7**, 525–537 (2011).

91. Bussi, G., Donadio, D. & Parrinello, M. Canonical sampling through velocity rescaling. *J. Chem. Phys.* **126**, 014101 (2007).

92. Parrinello, M. & Rahman, A. Polymorphic transitions in single crystals: A new molecular dynamics method. *Journal of Applied Physics* vol. 52 7182–7190 (1981).

93. Essmann, U. et al. A smooth particle mesh Ewald method. *The Journal of Chemical Physics* vol. 103 8577–8593 (1995).

94. Hess, B., Bekker, H., Berendsen, H. J. C. & Johannes G E. LINCS: A linear constraint solver for molecular simulations. *Journal of Computational Chemistry* vol. 18 1463–1472 (1997).

95. Yuan, C., Chen, H. & Kihara, D. Effective inter-residue contact definitions for accurate protein fold recognition. *BMC Bioinformatics* **13**, 292 (2012).

96. Trbovic, N. et al. Protein side-chain dynamics and residual conformational entropy. *J. Am. Chem. Soc.* **131**, 615–622 (2009).

97. Benson, N. C. & Daggett, V. A comparison of multiscale methods for the analysis of molecular dynamics simulations. *J. Phys. Chem. B* **116**, 8722–8731 (2012).

98. Chi, C. N. et al. Reassessing a sparse energetic network within a single protein domain. *Proc. Natl. Acad. Sci. U. S. A.* **105**, 4679–4684 (2008).

99. Johnson, Q. R., Lindsay, R. J., Nellas, R. B., Fernandez, E. J. & Shen, T. Mapping allostery through computational glycine scanning and correlation analysis of residue-residue contacts. *Biochemistry* **54**, 1534–1541 (2015).

100. Rasquinha, J. A., Bej, A., Dutta, S. & Mukherjee, S. Intrinsic Differences in Backbone Dynamics between Wild Type and DNA-Contact Mutants of the p53 DNA Binding Domain Revealed by Nuclear Magnetic Resonance Spectroscopy. *Biochemistry* **56**, 4962–4971 (2017).

101. D'Abramo, M. *et al.* The p53 tetramer shows an induced-fit interaction of the C-terminal domain with the DNA-binding domain. *Oncogene* **35**, 3272–3281 (2016).

102. Duan, J. & Nilsson, L. Effect of Zn2+ on DNA recognition and stability of the p53 DNA-binding domain. *Biochemistry* **45**, 7483–7492 (2006).

103. Bullock, A. N. *et al.* Thermodynamic stability of wild-type and mutant p53 core domain. *Proc. Natl. Acad. Sci. U. S. A.* **94**, 14338–14342 (1997).

104. Thukral, S. K., Blain, G. C., Chang, K. K. & Fields, S. Distinct residues of human p53 implicated in binding to DNA, simian virus 40 large T antigen, 53BP1, and 53BP2. *Mol. Cell. Biol.* **14**, 8315–8321 (1994).

105. Vijayabaskar, M. S. & Vishveshwara, S. Interaction Energy Based Protein Structure Networks. *Biophysical Journal* vol. 99 3704–3715 (2010).

106. Pagano, B. *et al.* Structure and stability insights into tumour suppressor p53 evolutionary related proteins. *PLoS One* **8**, e76014 (2013).

107. Li, Y. *et al.* Functional Diversity of p53 in Human and Wild Animals. *Front. Endocrinol.* **10**, 152 (2019).

108. Joo, W. S. *et al.* Structure of the 53BP1 BRCT region bound to p53 and its comparison to the Brca1 BRCT structure. *Genes Dev.* **16**, 583–593 (2002).

109. Butler, J. S. & Loh, S. N. Structure, function, and aggregation of the zinc-free form of the

p53 DNA binding domain. *Biochemistry* **42**, 2396–2403 (2003).

110. Joerger, A. C., Ang, H. C. & Fersht, A. R. Structural basis for understanding oncogenic p53 mutations and designing rescue drugs. *Proc. Natl. Acad. Sci. U. S. A.* **103**, 15056–15061 (2006).

111. Singh, S. *et al.* The cancer-associated, gain-of-function TP53 variant P152Lp53 activates multiple signaling pathways implicated in tumorigenesis. *J. Biol. Chem.* **294**, 14081–14095 (2019).

112. Okorokov, A. L. *et al.* The structure of p53 tumour suppressor protein reveals the basis for its functional plasticity. *EMBO J.* **25**, 5191-5200 (2006).

113. Mandal, A. K. *et al.* Glutamate counteracts the denaturing effect of urea through its effect on the denatured state. *J. Biol. Chem.* **278**, 36077–36084 (2003).

www.ingramcontent.com/pod-product-compliance
Lightning Source LLC
LaVergne TN
LVHW010600070526
838199LV00063BA/5020